UNDER THE DOCTOR

Studies in the psychological problems
of physiotherapists, patients and doctors

UNDER THE DOCTOR

Studies in the psychological problems
of physiotherapists, patients and doctors

Stanford Bourne

Avebury

First published in 1981 by Avebury Publishing Company, England.
© S. Bourne, 1981
All rights reserved.

British Library Cataloguing in Publication Data
Bourne, Stanford
  Under the doctor.
  1. Physical therapist and patient
  1. Title
  615′. 82′023   RM 701
  ISBN 0-86127-601-9

Printed and bound in Great Britain by
REDWOOD BURN LIMITED
Trowbridge & Esher

Contents

		Page
Author's note		7
Introduction		9
Part I	Observations arising from the sessions	13
	1 The Tavistock medical seminars	15
	2 The paramedical role	28
	3 The feminine professional image	34
	4 A remedial profession?	39
	5 Professional isolation	47
	6 The case history: enough or too much	52
	7 Anxieties and physical contact	57
	8 Mimicry and trickery	66
	9 Transcript of a seminar session	69
Part II	Session notes and cases	103
	Index of cases	188

5

Author's note

War brings out the best and the worst in people, and so does illness. As patients, doctors, nurses and physiotherapists struggle with illness and with each other, the situations that develop range from deeply moving tragedy and epic heroism to highly stylised comedy or plain farce.

Charming young physiotherapist: Keep at it, Mr Jenkins! We're going to put you in the Olympics next summer!

Grumpy old man on crutches: Piss off!

This report is dedicated to the physiotherapists who contributed to this study — they were superb. Professional discretion demands that they remain anonymous. Their reward shall be hereafter: in this life they will continue to be overlooked, underpaid and overworked. Theirs is a young profession.

The constant factor in this study is the idiocy of the doctor and the idealised awe employed to keep the poor man in his role. True, more and more women are doctors now and many physiotherapists are men. A very different book would result from a study of male physiotherapists and lady doctors, but this book is an account of the work of a group of women in a man's world.

Doctors suffer from their long history as quacks. Until one hundred years ago, no treatment at all was usually better than any existing treatment. Now that we can often cure people, we are like a bunch of conjurors and card-sharpers who suddenly find ourselves genuinely doing some of the things we have always pretended to do.

Doctors are the victims of their professional past, their patients, their colleagues — and, above all, of disease. This book is concerned with some of the ways that medical people are pushed and pulled into peculiar forms of behaviour. Most doctors know how often they must put up with being bad doctors; some of the best doctors die young, struggling to be good bad ones. As actuaries know, doctors have a raised susceptibility to coronary disease and to suicide — and this is even worse for psychiatrists.

My thanks to Murray Sperber for his generous editorial help.

The Tavistock Clinic, London, January 1980

7

Introduction

This book began as the report of an unusual and moving experience in a rather limited realm of medical education. When we began our work, we thought we might possibly be able to produce, not exactly a new textbook, but a rudimentary map of some landmarks and dangers in uncharted territory: a study of the psychological problems met by physiotherapists in the course of their work.

What is the physiotherapist to do when the patient insists he can't move a joint, yet she is sure he can? How is she to answer the patient who wants to know if he has cancer, when the doctor has said nothing? Suppose the consultant asks the physiotherapist to arrange for the patient's discharge from hospital: is it her job? And what if the doctor discharges her patient without asking her first: should this mean war? A young man has backache and wants to be massaged; another patient frequently makes the physiotherapist lose her temper.

It was soon apparent that physiotherapists often have more trouble with doctors and nurses than they have with difficult patients. We believe that our discoveries may be of equal interest to all members of the medical team in and out of hospital: this includes the oldest member of the team — the patient. The patient is the principal continuing factor shaping the character of the treatment he and his illness receive. If this book is readable, it is hoped that some patients will read it. We shall reach towards the concept of the-patient-as-colleague and hope that non-medical readers will enter into this area of interdisciplinary study.

Psychoanalysts are concerned constantly with the nature of the therapeutic alliance, the quest for that co-operating part of the patient who will join in promoting the analytic work. It may be part of the Apostolic Function of the psychoanalyst to seek out the nature of the therapeutic alliance in other areas of therapeutics. (The Apostolic Function of doctors is described later.) This is not merely a question of how to get patients to be co-operative — our shallow delight in the good patient: it is rather a matter of characterising the ambivalence in everyone and grappling with its

9

contradictions. Humans are hard to help.

A grim joke amongst doctors is that those patients for whom they have done most are rarely the most grateful — they are sometimes the angriest. Conversely, even the most good-natured and appreciative of patients are mystified at the thoughtless, inept and hurtful behaviour they so often encounter when they are ill, and especially when they go to hospital. This book tries to understand the thoughtless behaviour in the medical team; this includes some study of the kindness that killed the cat and various other failures of high hopes. We shall not merely be concerned with quarrels and complaints but more extensively with a range of many subtle and interesting problems — including a look at some solutions and puzzling successes.

We must enter and ventilate the shady psychological infra-structure of medical and para-medical behaviour, an area extensively disturbed by anxieties, rivalries, sexual feeling and much else. The patient, our first concern, is the casualty but the physiotherapist, the doctor, the nurse and the social worker may suffer injury too.

The findings and their connections will be new to many colleagues who are otherwise familiar with the concepts and methods employed and, to this extent, the book is quite advanced, requiring close reading at times. Nevertheless, it is also addressed to anybody interested in psychological and sociological matters, as well as to physiotherapists, doctors and nurses. It speaks to all those who wonder what goes on behind the bedside manners, good and bad, that patients encounter and especially to those who cherish the (vain?) hope that understanding may help. It is also intended, somewhat incidentally, to present a working exposition of applied psychoanalytic theory in relation to social systems. The material should enable the reader to examine the meaning of concepts such as transference, unconscious fantasy, part-objects, double-binds, etc., in terms of ordinary experience rather than as part of a scientific theology. A few key concepts are discussed and spelled out, as an unavoidable digression but, in the main, it is hoped that a direct style of presentation, free from technical jargon, may more accurately convey a sense of how the work was carried out. The best analytic work uses the simplest language.

The book is based upon the work of a group of physiotherapists who met weekly for about a year and a half to study the psychological aspects of their work, in a seminar led by a psychoanalyst at the Tavistock Clinic. Analogous seminars for doctors have been held at the Clinic for nearly 30 years and their example has had a world-wide influence on the training of doctors. Seminars for persons in other disciplines are also held but have not been publicly described in the same detail. At the beginning is a brief historical and theoretical introduction to the work of the Tavistock Clinic and the GP and Allied Professional Workshop within which the seminar was held.

Treatments involving numerous medical disciplines are often badly co-ordinated and hospital staff frequently seem to be evasive, thoughtless or arrogant. A central thesis evolves concerning the anxieties generated in medical staff by disease and death. The commonest defensive pattern is for doctors to tumble into postures of omnipotence whilst their non-medical colleagues are caught in complementary attitudes of angry subservience or fawning deference. Since most doctors are men while physiotherapists, nurses, radiographers, occupational therapists and hospital social workers are mostly women, the collusion is compounded and muddled by sexual roles, excitements and traditions. There are various other configurations in which the patient's treatment may become entangled but the seminar also shows physiotherapists capable of creative ingenuity in solving problems.

Part I presents the themes, observations and conclusions that arose from the seminar sessions. The text of Part I includes an annotated verbatim transcript of one session of the seminar. The session is of considerable dramatic interest as a story in its own right and also highlights some important theoretical and technical issues.

Part II presents the author's session summary notes made after each meeting of the seminar. Their publication should enable colleagues to re-examine their thoughts about styles and processes of leadership, teaching, study and research — as well as offering the reader an opportunity to evaluate the material upon which conclusions are based.

Part I

Observations arising from the sessions

Chapter 1

The Tavistock medical seminars

This seminar for physiotherapists (held between March 1972 and July 1973) was an activity of the GP and Allied Professional Workshop of the Tavistock Clinic. The Tavistock Clinic is an out-patient psychiatric clinic within the National Health Service in London. Founded in 1920 as an out-patient psychiatric clinic to provide treatment leavened by new psychoanalytic and sociological insights, it developed into a unique national institution. The Tavistock Clinic, together with its sister organisation, the Tavistock Institute of Human Relations, has become a national centre for training and research in psychotherapy and for the application of psychological understanding into work lying beyond traditional psychiatry — into medicine, 'the helping professions', and the fabric of society itself. The basic work of the Clinic remains the treatment of the individual patient and his family but, apart from many formal courses, important consultative work is carried out with such people as probation officers, teachers, industrial managers, government employees, airline personnel, etc., a clientele reflecting the larger concerns of community mental health and illness.

The GP and Allied Professional Workshop is one of many enclaves of activity within the Tavistock Clinic and is the development of the celebrated work with general practitioners started by Dr Michael Balint[1] in 1951. The Workshop's concepts and ingredients (and it is like a mixture of religion, science and cookery) come from psychoanalysis, group therapy, group dynamics and the social preoccupations of the Tavistock's 50-year history, together with the inspiration of Michael Balint and some 30 years of discussion amongst his colleagues and successors.

Dr Balint first became interested in the psychological problems of family doctors with their patients as a young man in Hungary before the war. When

[1] Michael Balint, 1896—1970. Born Budapest, son of a GP. Came to England as refugee in 1939. Psychoanalyst, psychiatrist, writer and innovator.

he began seminars on the subject at the Tavistock Clinic in 1951 there was an intense interest at the Clinic in group therapy and group processes. During the war certain leading British psychoanalysts[1] in the Army had applied group interests and theories to problems of officer-selection and the rehabilitation of war neurosis, repatriated prisoners of war etc. Balint's personal interest in the psychology of general practice came to be studied therefore in an institution where there was considerable sophistication in the use and study of groups; and this knowledge of groups was already being applied to seminar teaching in various areas of related work. Outside the Clinic, the scene was dominated by the recent inception in 1948 of the National Health Service which had transformed the work of British doctors.

The general practitioner seminars

When Balint started his first seminar in 1951 he struck gold. General practice in Britain was ready for a renaissance and the influence of these seminars was one of the biggest single factors in the revival that followed. Surveys were beginning to demonstrate that at least one-third of patients calling on their GPs were suffering from undisguised psychological problems, while an unknown proportion of the remainder had illnesses and disturbances with a large psychological component. In the context of the new National Health Service and in a new era of scientific medicine, GPs confronting these psychological problems were losing their self-respect. Aware of their total lack of training in psychology, they tended to react with angry helplessness, as well as guilt and resentment towards these patients who were 'wasting their time'. Formerly, the patient died with the old family doctor sitting by the bedside through the night whereas now, the patient's life was saved by a young man whose name he didn't quite catch.

Balint applied his attention to the psychological problems in general practice, and showed how they might be studied creatively, at precisely the time when this development was desperately needed. Unless GPs could regain a fundamental self-respect throughout their work, it was impossible to maintain proper standards, even in the more physical side of the work — and the Collings Report[2] had shocked everybody with its revelations. By the 1970s the standard of general practice in Britain never stood higher; there is a Royal College of General Practitioners, professors of general practice teach in the medical schools and Vocational Training Schemes for general practice are becoming mandatory. Participation in so-called

---

[1] W R Bion, H Bridger, H Ezriel, S H Foulkes, T F Main, J Rickman and J D Sutherland amongst others.
[2] J S Collings, 'General Practice in England Today', *Lancet*, 1950, Vol I, pp. 555–585.

16

'Balint Groups' are often an obligatory feature of these training programmes.

An International Balint Society was started in Europe after Balint's death in 1970. At the Tavistock Clinic, we prefer to speak of GP seminars rather than Balint Groups, in the hope of avoiding the implication of a theology with only one received way of doing things. Indeed, we arrange for GPs in seminars to work with different seminar leaders after two years; this combats any tendency to settle into a comfortable arrangement of mutual blind spots.

Seminars meet one afternoon a week (excepting school holidays) for years on end. There is no curriculum or syllabus and the work is based on the GPs' experience with their patients. Cases are discussed and data examined with the 'third ear' of the psychoanalyst and a sense of the seminar's own group dynamics; the seminar leader's understanding of the group dynamic may often tell him more about the problem than any other evidence. The situation in the seminars tends to reflect and mimic the clinical problems preoccupying its members. The central point of reference in the examination of each story is the doctor-patient relationship, its evolution and handling and its bearing on the management of the case. The seminar members come to know each other closely and it is part of the responsibility of leadership to ensure that the intimacy does not degenerate into the atmosphere of a club, where the hard work would be submerged. It is the task of the seminar to clarify the professional profile of each doctor as well as to dissect the problem in each case presented. Strengths and weaknesses become exposed and there is time for doctors to experiment towards their own professional development, with the critical support of the seminar at hand. There is an atmosphere of discovery and development, in a research team with its leader.

It became recognisable that different doctors have their own various ways of establishing a language of symptoms and treatments with different patients and that this plays a big part in determining the character of 'the illness', upon which the doctor and patient agree to settle. This might be a compromise between different physical, psychological and social preoccupations and pressures in the patient's life, as well as various predilections to which the doctor may be prone. Balint described the 'Apostolic Function' of doctors, in steering the patients' symptoms into specific directions. Formerly, the ordinary doctor was perceived as a rather passive technician, doing his best with the tasks placed before him. Doctors who were missionaries, researchers and reformers were the exceptions, like mutations. Now it has been recognised that all doctors influence patterns of disease (not just fashions of diagnosis), modes of symptom-presentation and the expectations and habits of their patients. Of course, some illnesses have an inexorable and calamitous momentum of their own: the doctor may be able to do little besides wringing his hands (or — to anticipate —

17

prescribing physiotherapy). We all owe Nature a death but, until the time comes, our transactions with the doctor are liable to have an à la carte configuration, with everything depending on what is chosen, from what is on offer. And the choosing is a bilateral process, with options on both sides.

It has long been known that the most potent item in the pharmacopoeia is the doctor himself. These seminars re-established serious attention to the pharmacology and use of the drug 'doctor'.

The central concern of the seminars is the nature of the doctor-patient relationship, and its bearing on the management and development of each case. A further concern of the seminars is the hope that the doctors might become better doctors, more flexible in their work and more contented in it — although this is never achieved without strain and pain. The notion of the seminar as a therapeutic group is strictly excluded (doctors requiring therapy have to seek it elsewhere) but the work done and the skills gained could result eventually in 'a limited but considerable change in the doctor'. This is one of the phrases which Balint coined and it was a lucky stroke that, like most celebrated scientific pioneers, he could not only make advances in knowledge but had the gift of being able to write about them vividly. His book, *The Doctor, His Patient and the Illness*, has been translated into French, German, Hungarian, Italian and Spanish.

The Tavistock GP and Allied Professional Workshop

When Balint started his GP Seminars in the 1950s, the Tavistock already had behind it thirty years work with teachers, social workers, probation officers etc who struggled with psychological problems in other people. Balint's work with the GP came to carry his indelible stamp but the vitality of the work also depended, in a considerable degree, on differing viewpoints regarding the techniques and styles of seminar leadership. An energetic forum for the study of this field of work came into existence with regular meetings to discuss techniques of leading seminars. Particular effort was given to the study of verbatim transcripts, which were analysed and debated into the night at meetings held in Michael and Enid Balint's house. Part of this book is devoted to the verbatim transcript of one session of the physiotherapists' seminar. A number of Balint's colleagues at the Tavistock Clinic were particularly interested in group therapy and a wider study of group process as well as the application of GP seminar experience to work with other disciplines.

In 1967, a group of colleagues published a collection of papers setting out some of the thinking behind these later developments in the work.[1]

---

[1] *The Use of Small Groups in Training*, R Gosling, D H Miller, D Woodhouse and P M Turquet (Codicote Press, London, 1967).

After his retirement from the NHS, Balint continued work with GPs and with medical students at University College Hospital. Dr T F Main, at the Cassel Hospital, has played a leading role in the development of psychological skills in doctors working in family planning clinics, specialising in contraceptive techniques but also constantly confronting sexual and matrimonial problems. At the Tavistock, there have been seminars for dentists, clergy, nurses, health visitors, factory doctors, probation officers, social workers — and now, physiotherapists. It will be noticed that, in some of these professions, there is little or none of the opportunity for practising either 'counselling' or 'straight psychotherapy' which some GPs can make a considerable part of their job. This underlines the ethos of the GP and Allied Professional Workshop in its endeavour to delineate the transference processes and to develop psychological skills appropriate for the separate professions — a very different matter from teaching other professionals to do psychotherapy. In spite of any parallel hope that GPs may develop skill in psychotherapy for neurotic problems, the central concern of the Workshop is that they may be able to improve their psychological skill as doctors, skill in handling every type of medical contingency, including the anxieties around birth and death as well as disease.

The GP and Allied Professional Workshop embraces this whole range of seminars but the practical sense in which it is a workshop depends on the regular meetings of seminar leaders and associate leaders, to discuss the work and the training of new leaders.

There are certain essential features that characterise the seminars held within the GP and Allied Professional Workshops. The seminar leader is a practising psychoanalyst or at any rate, someone versed in psychoanalytic experience. He is also an experienced group therapist. He understands that he cannot teach the members of the seminars how to do their jobs. Hence, these seminars are very different from ordinary teaching seminars in which pupils gather with a tutor who has a clear onus to know his subject better than his pupils. Here it is a question more of leadership, steering a working group towards the most fruitful achievement of its tasks. There may be times when their work — collecting a history, discussing the patient's (or 'client's') anxieties with him, may be similar to the work of a psychoanalyst or psychiatrist. At that point it is very easy for the seminar leader to slide into the role of psychiatric teacher — and some leaders and seminar members believe we should do this more often.

The special skills of the psychoanalyst and the climate in which he nourishes these skills, can be a positive encumbrance when he has to adjust his sights towards fruitful work with other professions. Psychiatrists and psychoanalysts joining seminars as new associates immediately want to understand and interpret material events, constantly explaining and translating them, whereas they have to grasp the fact that many of these allied

professionals achieve their ends in an uncomprehending context of concrete
activity, physical contact and tacit exchanges. The GP's decisions whether
to visit, or whether to examine, or whether to touch, represent action which
speaks as loudly as psychoanalytical words. Psychoanalysts rarely advise
their patients what to do (although, of course, patients are influenced by
the interpretations they receive) and their physical contact with patients is
confined to the occasional shaking of hands, a few times a year. Members
of the other healing and helping professions have every kind of varied access
to their patients including frequent intimate physical contact. Doctors in
family planning clinics have discovered great possibilities in the exploration
of feelings and thoughts during vaginal examinations and can achieve
remarkable short cuts.

Training or treatment?

If a seminar is to delve into the psychological problems of professional work
it is inevitably carried into territory which may easily be mistaken for
personal psychotherapy for the members of the seminar. As they get to
know each other, the members of the seminar cultivate an impressive acute-
ness of hearing for each other's professional strengths and weaknesses, as
well as their personal quirks. This is usually achieved within an atmosphere
of keen attentiveness leavened by some humour. Of course, blindness still
abounds and, without it, the seminar would have no work to do. For that
matter, the seminar would probably be unable to continue if its members
were not able, from time to time, to switch their blindness on and off, as
anxieties demand.

Strangely enough, intense anxieties and disturbances have a tendency to
emerge more during the very early sessions than they do afterwards. At
first, alarms and intimacies come tumbling out but later the seminar becomes
somewhat guarded. Thus, we learn in the second session that a close relative
of one member has a serious illness – a distinctly awkward piece of personal
information. In the third session we are presented with a patient who is also
a member of the seminar's own profession – a physiotherapist.

There is always a special sigh of relief when the treatment of a professional colleague goes according to plan, for such cases have a knack of going
wrong on a scale rarely matched with other patients. There is, similarly,
an extra element of perpexity for a seminar presented with the case of a
professional colleague as patient. Such a case always stirs the suspicion that
it will present problems that are more personal than the average case, more
likely to reveal us as patients ourselves. If they are not quite as we ourselves
are, they are uncomfortably like brothers and sisters to us. In the third
meeting of the sessions reported in detail later, Ms Ash presents the case of
a physiotherapist (Case No 6) and has actually been driven to beg her to
'forget that she had ever been a physiotherapist'. The discussion is continued

in the next session and, indeed, reappears throughout the life of the seminar, the case being eventually taken over by one of her colleagues.

Cases presented in pairs are often linked in ways that may become apparent to an alert seminar. In the fourth session Ms Ash's addendum to the first case is linked with the case of another young woman (Case No 7) of totally different type — supposedly. However, it is soon mentioned in passing that this next patient's brother is a doctor — so there is still a central preoccupation with the patient who is within the professional family and is possibly our twin. Ms Ash demonstrates the skilled use of selective blindness in this case as she decides that it would be best not to know about the patient's row with the previous physiotherapist — judging, accurately, that discussing rows may not be her forte. We can further see the problem of the physiotherapist-as-patient showing through, in the shape of this anonymous predecessor. The seminar colluded with Ms Ash in drawing a veil over her views about this cblleague: we are, at this stage, still not sure how far we are discussing the psychological problems of patients and how far we are to go in discussing the psychological problems of staff — ultimately, the problems of the physiotherapists themselves that will certainly become discernable in the here-and-now of the seminars.

The agreed policy and theory is fairly easy to state but often hard to delineate and apply in practice. The seminar should study, to the limit of its ability, the *professional* habits, strengths and weakness of its members and yet avoid the intrusion of private and personal difficulties from becoming an illegitimate field of attention.

A seminar of this type has to struggle with problems of intimacy and distance. These reflect similar issues that are encountered in work with patients. It might seem that greater intimacy and familiarity should lead to a growth of trust, honesty and co-operation. This view disregards common experience although it may follow a current tendency towards over-valuation of openness, communication and the abolition of barriers. This trend is related to the spirit of the times but it is, more specifically, a direct result of misapplied psychoanalytic insights. Since Freud demonstrated that so much neurosis was due to unconscious conflict and since so much of the work of psychoanalysis involves rendering unconscious thought into conscious insight, there is liable to be an unwarranted assumption that it is always best to bring things into the open. Actually, to understand all is not necessarily to forgive all and honesty is not always the best policy. This is what tact and diplomacy are about but the matter goes further than that.

The problem has to do with the security of frontiers and the desirable strength of barriers. The psychological problem resembles the territorial one. The ideal condition is for a frontier to be so strong and secure that there will be no arguments and fights over it but, at the same time, there should be the greatest possible freedom for movement backwards and forwards across it. It is a matter of strength with suppleness. The mind has an unhappy tendency to develop rigidity with brittleness. The work of psychoanalysis is not merely to make the unconscious conscious but, more important, to strengthen mental organisation and flexibility and achieve a healthy flux between the inner world and outer reality.

In its early stages, a seminar is likely to swing between awkward shyness, wary evasiveness (and healthy caution), and impulsive and embarrassing disclosures. The early work of the seminar is to establish necessary habits of organisation and style so that a real and working intimacy can develop. A seminar requires at least a year or two before it has forged a reliable structure of knowledge and trust within which exploration can extend so that its members can cope effectively with their discoveries. It means living through disappointment and disillusion, after the early excitement.

Tape-recorders and privacy

We now tape-record all seminars in the GP and Allied Professional Workshop in case we wish to study the material further and also to establish tape-recording as a routine. We thereby avoid the excessive disturbance that would be caused by introducing a tape-recorder at a later stage, if it should be specifically required. The tapes are erased and re-used later on, unless specially required. All the tapes of the physiotherapists' seminar were kept and this was made clear to the members of the seminar. In view of the intimacy and honesty that develops in the course of this work, the tapes are locked away as highly confidential material, and they are transcribed only by reliable secretaries of known integrity and loyalty. Transcripts have pseudonyms substituted for real names and places.

The principal problems are not ones of technique and organisation. Experience forces us to recognise that all sorts of persecutory anxiety and guilt are stirred, on every side, by the endeavour to record live conversations.

The problems and anxieties around confidentiality, intrusiveness, exhibitionism and voyeurism, interfere in the relationship between patients and the people looking after them. That is why the foregoing discussion is not a tangential digression but, on the contrary, an attempt to thrust towards the heart of the matter. So much of what we regard as neutral, conflict-free, 'not a problem' (a favourite claim of seminar members reluctant to describe their work) is fraught with anguish and embarrassment of which we are liable to have very little conscious inkling.

Transference, counter-transference and the relationship with patients

Freud was slow to discover transference and counter-transference in psycho-analytic work seventy years ago, so perhaps it is not odd that it took so long before anyone began systematically to study their ramifications in other medical situations. Psychoanalysis nearly foundered, at the outset, from transference problems. Freud's colleague Breuer, in their early work on hysteria,[1] became profoundly alarmed by the attachment one of his patients developed for him. Breuer's own marriage was threatened as the case came to command more and more of his emotional energy. Breuer bowed out over this eventually, as well as from his reluctance to associate himself with Freud's discoveries of sexual trauma and sexual fantasy, behind hysteria. At first, Freud thought that all these patients had been sexually molested in childhood and, in spite of the fury he aroused, he insisted on publishing these findings. Later, he realised that what he had discovered was the extent of sexual fantasy behind hysteria and the compelling force of unconscious imagination; the psychic reality of fantasy life may shape subjective experience and personality development equally with the actual experiences of real life.

Transference is a technical term referring to a specific expression of a universal process. Transference is not merely an affair of psychoanalytic patients either loving or hating the analyst. Neither is it a question of the patient going through stages of seeing the analyst as the incarnation of his mother, father or family. In fact, we all experience our world, subjectively, according to the way we invest it with unconscious beliefs, expectations, fears and wishes — all of which interact constantly with the actual stimuli and perceptions we receive from the things and people existing around us. There is a tremendous valency or gravitation towards perception of other people in the light of images from the past. These figures, present, external, 'real' objects, together with internalised images from the past, are all con-ceived in the light of our own projections, the features we imagine and impute. Hence, one person is never seen in quite the same way by any two others and our present experience of the people in our lives is governed by the state of our inner worlds; and these, in turn, are archives of past experience, forgotten passions together with all our current needs and urges.

Each patient experiences the analyst in his own way, which changes all the time; and the dissection of this conscious and unconscious experience of the analyst, in all its modality, is what we mean by analysis of the trans-ference.[2] It is in the nature of things, and to be expected, that analogous

---

[1] Breuer and Freud, *Studies On Hysteria*, 1895.
[2] Counter-transference is the corresponding configuration of fact, fancy and prejudice which add up to the psychoanalyst's experience of his patient.

processes of transference - a mixture of echo and projections – occur in relationships in which important aspects of infantile experience are repeated. This is particularly the case in relation to people like teachers and doctors, people in authority and people to whom we can relate in an infantile sort of way. Most of us are liable to feel very small indeed when we go to hospital as patients and regression tends to be encouraged by everything in the situation and, especially, by being put to bed and nursed.

Transference is unconscious.
There are dimensions to these matters which tend to be easily overlooked. Firstly, some of the most compelling emotional transferences from the past, onto present objects, remain totally unconscious. Transference is not merely an obvious matter of falling in love with the doctor or feeling like a baby in the hands of the nurse. It is subtle, fragmentary, fleeting, and this helps to explain why patients are sometimes mercurial and bewildering in the way they change their attitudes towards hospital staff. The patient, on his side, may be equally bewildered, feeling swept up in feelings or nuances of mood that are as unexpected as they are disturbing.

Transference and part-objects.
Another difficult feature of transference phenomena, stemming from infantile sources, is that so many of the feelings and attitudes are concerned with part-objects rather than whole people. Part-object relationships mean, to the psychoanalyst, that the person views and experiences bits of other people and bits of his world as if they were whole people with their own autonomy. The baby probably experiences the breast or the nipple as an entity capable of sustaining an independent relationship and animated by a range of feelings and impulses attributed to it on the basis of actual experience and on the basis of projection. It is a familiar observation that people are sometimes inclined to treat other people as 'things', usually a sign of the strange world of part-object relationships, often weird but passing for normal.

The doctor and the physiotherapist encounter the reverse side of the process, the side that is less obvious socially – although obvious enough in the vicissitudes of sexual life – whereby the organs of the body are anthropomorphised, invested with autonomous human and inhuman animation. Some of the greatest disturbances in the doctor-patient or physiotherapist-patient relationships, arise from the way they share deeply disturbing beliefs and fears about the organs of the body. Part-object relationships involving appliances and gadgets arise particularly easily because these can be so difficult to place, psychologically. Orthopaedic appliances, the marvels of medical gadgetry, and, above all, the weirdness of artificial limbs, can all be deeply disturbing and confusing, even to quite stable people.

24

Some of these processes can be discerned in Ms Mahogany's Case No 21 where the patient's perception of the physiotherapist and the relationship with her were confused with complex feelings about the knee. The unexpected loss of the patella ('losing her bits and bobs') is merged with the recent loss of the mother (by death). Possibly the surgical mutilation reactivates the primitive anxieties about family and body, comprising what analysts see as 'separation enxiety' and 'castration anxiety'. The patient has no trust or optimism in developing the power of her quadriceps muscles to compensate for the double and merged loss (patella and mother). Her behaviour is deeply puzzling to the physiotherapist as her anxiety appears to be out of all proportion to the ostensible mechanics of an unstable knee and the need for quadriceps drill to secure it. She desperately wants the physiotherapist to hold her leg for her; the knee is like her baby-self, who needs mother to hold her securely. She wants the physiotherapist to become mother, but in a way that is very specific and related to preoccupations about bodily parts and their disappearance, rather than in the more general way in which the mother might be missed and mourned as a real person.

The physiotherapists' seminar

A local branch of the Chartered Society of Physiotherapy invited the author to give a talk describing the work of GP seminars at the Tavistock Clinic. But then we agreed that it would be more interesting if there could be a similar seminar for physiotherapists and if the work of that seminar could be presented to the meeting. The GP seminars continue for a period of several years and this horizon of work enables intimacy and trust to develop giving the doctors time to experiment, reflect and develop – and to discover themselves. This was clearly going to be impossible to set up overnight with the physiotherapists but we decided, nevertheless, to try to capture some flavour of the GP seminar work. A notice went out to departments of physiotherapy in some hospitals around London to enlist members for an experimental seminar. Ten physiotherapists came forward and we held our first session on 1 March 1972. We agreed to have four weekly sessions of one and a half hours each and then to consider how best we might present ourselves to the quarterly meeting of their Society. After these four sessions there was the possibility that I, as leader of the seminar, might attempt to report our experience or this might be done as a combined venture. However, the seminar seemed to go well and we felt strong enough to try out a different possibility.

Some large rooms at the Tavistock Clinic are equipped with two-way mirror observation screens so that the proceedings in one room may be watched by an audience of observers in an adjacent room. This is never done without the knowledge and consent of the people who are being observed. It is simply that it is easier to forget about the audience if they are not visible and, thereby, distraction and distortion from self-consciousness are minimised. So, for the quarterly meeting, we held a session of the seminar on our own in one room, whilst being observed by the remaining members of the meeting in the next room. There were perhaps twenty-five observers. We reduced the session from our normal hour and a half to one hour, in order to leave time for an introduction beforehand and a full discussion together afterwards.

The evening went very successfully: the session was intensely interesting, we gave a fair representation of ourselves at work — given due allowance for the loss of intimacy. The discussion afterwards was fruitful and stimulating. Following upon this event, I shared the enthusiasm to continue, expressed by some members of the seminar and certain of the observers who were interested in joining. There was a difficulty over the time factor. Psycho-analysts are used to thinking of treatments that continue for several years and they have been personally committed, in their training, to a personal analysis that goes on even longer than most of their patients' treatments. On the other hand, most hospital doctors and (especially) surgeons are used to working within the time-scale of acute illness and in the pressure of overcrowded wards and waiting-lists. Only very exceptional medical people find it easy to attune to the pace and perspective of psychoanalysts, used to waiting years for important but subtle changes. As a compromise, we decided to plan a seminar for one year — the maximum that might be accepted by their colleagues and seniors, if physiotherapists working in hospital departments were to be given leave to attend.

The seminar reconvened some weeks later — after Easter 1972. There were five members of the original seminar (of ten people) and one new member. We were later joined by three more people; and we were also re-joined, for a time, by one more of the original band. We were able to continue until the summer holiday, which gave us four terms in all. Altogether, we had 51 meetings.

All the members of the seminar were women and we had to decide whether to accept this as a lopsided arrangement which reflected a lop-sided profession. At different times, two men did express interest in joining but there was the impression that their working situations were very different from the others in the seminar and it seemed best to continue what we were doing rather than attempting to cover everything.

These women were not a random sample of physiotherapists and certain exceptional qualities and strengths as well as anxieties impelled them to join the seminar. Nonetheless, they appeared to be a remarkably normal bunch of people. They were all seasoned in their work, many occupying positions of senior responsibility though half were youngsters in their 20s and the others ranged into middle-age. The work and cases studied were fairly typical of the ordinary problems most physiotherapists encounter in their daily work with the average run of patients.

We met one afternoon each week, excepting school holidays. The sessions were for one and a half hours and were all tape-recorded. The proceedings were based entirely upon the open invitation to members of the seminar, 'Who has a case?'[1] Cases would then be presented according to the pressure that different people were experiencing, rather than in any set order. This is reflected in the list of cases presented by each member of the seminar (see the Appendix). Some preferred to focus on a few cases and would probably have preferred more open discussions of general topics. However, in this Workshop we are convinced of the necessity to attach discussion to specific chapter and verse, being otherwise left in the realms of prejudice, fantasy, bluff and mutual admiration. Moreover, the presentation of an account of actual work gets much closer to the real anxieties involved than a general discussion would do. Further, only in focussing on actual cases do the unconscious problems emerge.

[1] The extensive meaning and implications underlying this seemingly simple way of opening is discussed at length by Gosling and Turquet, p. 50 of *The Uses Of Small Groups In Training* (Codicote Press & Tavistock Institute of Human Relations, 1967).

Chapter 2

The paramedical role

The patient is often hurt in the crossfire between the groups of assorted professionals who look after him. This partly explains the relative impotence of associations seeking to protect the patient from the hospital. The patient would be better helped if the doctors, nurses, and administrators could be protected from one another.

A separate book could be written about the relationship between physiotherapists and doctors, and it is hard sometimes to avoid the impression that physiotherapists are more oppressed by problems with doctors than they ever are by problems with patients. Physiotherapists are included together with a number of other professional groups designated, rather unhappily, as the 'paramedical professions'. Another term that has been used is 'professions ancillary to medicine'. The extent to which they are meant to be handmaidens of the Lord is an agonising issue.

Physiotherapists have to work within the sanction of the doctor and the meaning of this sanction can vary enormously. The physiotherapist may be required to execute the doctor's prescription of treatment in minute detail or she may work as a virtually independent practitioner to whom the doctor refers the patient, as to another specialist. There is nothing to stop any lay person offering their unsupervised services in a sauna bath or via a postcard in a newsagent's shop-window, but a trained physiotherapist who wishes to remain on the professional register does not treat patients without the sanction of a doctor.

The professional requirement that the physiotherapist work within the sanction of the doctor'tends to spread like a miasma and there is sometimes the impression that she is not supposed to use her head at all. Occasionally, the physiotherapist is found valiantly maintaining that black is white, if that is what the doctor is supposed to have said. It may become difficult for the physiotherapist to recover and re-assert her independence of mind without swinging over into a belligerent or petulant defiance that she

28

knows, simultaneously, to be quite inappropriate and unnecessary.

She relapses into stifled resentment. The entire cycle of events is displayed very clearly in Case 62 (28th February, 14th and 28th March, 1973). Professional deference to the doctor may keep him hopelessly uninformed and behaving with fatuous ineffectiveness — and this may keep the patient incapacitated too. More subtle aspects of the problem are seen, for example, in Case 38 (8th and 22nd November, 1972), where a posture of gentle femininity and compliance left a man helpless on his back.

Subservience to the doctor is not always adopted in a climate of idealisation and it is, of course, often resented bitterly; and idealisation itself is not an innocent affair, simply a matter of admiration multiplied a few times over. It is not just a case of, 'My daddy is bigger than your daddy!': psychoanalysts know that idealisation is liable to veil hostility, contempt and anxiety about an object that has previously been injured and brought low; idealisation may also be placatory, in relation to an object that is threatening or frightening. In this sense, the state of the object, idealised, damaged, menacing or whatever, is rooted in the fantasy life of the subject — and may be totally different in real life.

In private practice, the physiotherapist may work in a fairly independent way even though conforming to correct professional etiquette. In hospital, independence is more restricted by the prevailing social structure, departmental hierarchies and local traditions. Few hospitals have yet managed to disencumber themselves from a past in which the consultant was a Prince of the Church, nurses were as lay nuns and physiotherapists did not exist. The social structures have changed but the same attitudes persist and this is another prime cause of chaotic staff behaviour.

Like nurses, physiotherapists are ridden with hierarchies and authority. These problems are no longer matters of individual psychopathology but are cemented into the management system of physiotherapy departments in hospitals. Ideally, a seminar at the Tavistock Clinic should not reflect these patterns. The seminar leader should avoid the role of bossy doctor and should try to defuse the hatred seething in the physiotherapeutic breast. There was, nevertheless, an insidious and relentless unconscious pressure to push the leader into this role of bossy know-all. Again and again we saw, in the cases reported in the seminar, the secret triumph of the physiotherapist over the idiot-doctor and the conspiracy to keep him that way; a seminar leader rides the same tiger and is never so worried as when all the seminar appear to agree with him.

The conflict was set forth unmistakably in the very first session — our first case. The physiotherapist's supervisor had 'very helpfully' gone over her lists with her, to pick out some 'suitable' patients to present at the seminar. (The physiotherapist was an experienced mature person but very ready to assume this subservient dependent role.) The patient selected had been referred from doctor to doctor whilst the physiotherapists, carrying out treatment, were unable to get the doctors to recognise the psychological problem they sensed. In our discussion there was firstly and crucially a supplication for the seminar leader to pronounce whether this was or was not 'a suitable case' for the seminar. Secondly, there were torrents of bitter complaints about the hopeless problem of wresting status and independence from the grasp of wilfully blind doctors. The ambivalent forces are transparent. The physiotherapists complain bitterly about the stupid boss-doctor and yet they beg the only doctor in the room to start bossing them around and telling them what to think. The seminar leader had already specified very clearly, at the outset, that he had no idea what they were going to discuss, or what they should discuss, and that the work of the seminar would be based on *their* professional experience, what *they* chose to report and thence to the invariable opening: 'Who has a case?'

In the case-history presented, the physiotherapists left the doctors in complacent ignorance as, supposedly, they 'have to obey' the medical prescription, however misconceived.[1] But what of the secret withering contempt? Significantly, the patient in the case was an adolescent girl adopted by a couple who, in their male-and-female roles, probably reflect the doctor-physiotherapist couple in important and uncomfortable ways. Like the spontaneous material the patient brings to mind in a psychoanalytic session, the cases chosen for mention in a seminar, and the particular slant they are given, are all liable to reflect the pattern of underlying preoccupations, and not merely the daily chance occurrences. Thus, the mother in the case displays a futile elegance whilst the father has a coronary thrombosis. The doctor-seminar-leader is invited to place his foot right on the banana skin too, by presuming to tell these experienced women what is a 'suitable' case to discuss. This background pattern, with its partnership of the immaculate woman and the man who dies of the strain, should be a warning to doctors who will always be faced with crucifixion and an early death, if they are deceived into playing God. The problem for the doctor is to live up to his elaborate training and his ultimate medical responsibilities without falling into delusions of omnipotence. It is often his job 'to know best' but he must avoid omniscience.

The same struggle probably continued throughout the life of the seminar and we could never escape completely from the delusion that the seminar leader might (as a doctor) know better than the members what was a psychological problem *to them* and, thence, what might be 'a suitable case' to discuss. Of course, there are leadership problems in any seminar. There are always decisions to be taken about how far to go in a discussion or when to turn to something else or, maybe, when to postpone a topic until the

---

[1] Other instances in which physiotherapists collude to leave the doctor ill-informed or misguided are Cases 62 and 63. By contrast, Case 67 shows how effective the physiotherapist may occasionally be in elucidating a muddle.

following week. The seminar leader must decide the scope he allows himself in actually voicing his own views and reactions. These technical problems of leadership are generically different from the enormous pressure upon the seminar leader to act in an omniscient way, to tell a group of people from an allied profession whether the psychological problems they experience in their jobs are 'suitable' to look at. It is in the nature of things that *after* the problem has been studied it may wear a different appearance and an important part of the seminar leader's work is to enable members of the seminar to recognise the disturbance emanating from problems of which they had not previously been conscious. In that particular sense there is some validity in the notion of telling people when they have a problem — suitable or not!

The 'paramedical' role, designated as a kind of appendage of somebody else, is conducive to a love-hate situation, a relationship of intense ambivalence. We have considered something of the way idealisation may conceal hostility and ridicule but, for much of the day, work is reasonably successful and co-operation with medical colleagues is uneventful and, quite often, rewarding. The orientation of the seminar's work around the examination of problems and anxieties can allow us to lose sight of some of the satisfactions — even delights — of hospital work. Many hospital doctors are very able people and, in their professional work, can display admirable qualities. The doctor is usually and genuinely, a key person in the treatment. Aside from the problems created by negative feelings about medical authority there are serious difficulties which stem from the positive feelings.

One untoward result of positive regard for admirable doctors may be the total and indiscriminate emulation of them — swallowing medical mores whole. Anybody who is expected to treat illness is under intense pressure to assume some of the styles and titles of omnipotence, but it is also possible to become *plus royaliste que le roi*. Thus, for example, we find physiotherapists transfixed by the belief that it is always necessary to appear poised, informed, confident. 'You must never appear uncertain in front of your patient'. 'You can never do any good with a patient who doesn't like you.' 'I couldn't let the patient see that I didn't know what the doctor had said.' Some of the most important work done in the seminar was the exploration and erosion of these paralysing tenets of faith.[1]

Worship of the doctor may work in the service of evasiveness. One compensation of a junior or subordinate position is that it allows you to seek support from seniors and for responsibility to be shared, or even passed on altogether. Beyond these legitimate bounds and beyond the appropriate

---

[1] We shall return to this issue — the quest for omnipotence — with added force in the discussion of chronic and incurable illness, on page 39.

deference to authority (which some people find so painful), there is another kind of deliberate defensive posturing behind vagueness and the skilled avoidance of knowing awkward facts. This is a story that repeats itself *ad nauseam* in the diary of the seminar — and in the daily hospital scene.

A number of aspects of a typical situation are displayed in Case 3. In this case the physiotherapist is an attractive young woman just married. The patient is a woman in her 30s who has just had a breast removed for cancer. The problem presented to the seminar is that she had been trans-ferred to Ms Ash by the Head of the Physiotherapy Department, owing to an unexplained quarrel with a previous physiotherapist. The patient asked Ms Ash whether she knew about the row and whether she wanted to know about it. At this point, it was most refreshing for a psychiatrist to observe Ms Ash free from the medical and psychiatric mores that can so easily take possession of a seminar like this. Whereas many doctors and most psychia-trists would have felt no option but to allow the patient to talk as she wished, Ms Ash firmly suggested that it might be best if they tried to start off afresh without going into all that. Instead, she turned to an examina-tion of the scar of the recent operation, and was glad to be able to admire it. It was, indeed, a very good, neat, clean scar. Here we see the intuitive behaviour of a person who knows what she can do well and what she cannot. She would not have been good at looking at the scar of the row with her colleague but she could somehow strike the right note by relying on her expertise as a physiotherapist. Thereupon, freed by this deft touch, the patient proceeded to ask about the diagnosis and prognosis, which she had not been told. But at this, the physiotherapist dived swiftly behind the doctor. Adopting a much more infantile role, she can lodge herself behind the question of, 'What did your doctor say?', as she herself, like the patient, has skilfully avoided acquiring any detailed information about the condition and the prognosis. Strikingly, the seminar too, contrived skilfully to discuss the situation for half an hour without actually exposing these thorny points, until the seminar leader chose to make himself awkward.

There is a tremendous pressure to fall in with the policy that it is better not to know, and that nobody really *has* to know anything, until the doctor takes it upon himself to make people know. The doctor works for his living in all sorts of ways and he very often does have to live up to his responsibility for taking decisions, for being clever if not wise. But we shall see later that there is a *quid pro quo* in some of the situations around serious illness (especially if there is also a significant social problem) when the doctor has an army of 'paramedical' women to bear his troubles.

In this area of feigned ignorance, or assumed ignorance elaborately maintained, the physiotherapist is in an especially awkward position, compared with doctors and nurses. The nurse (and particularly the junior nurse) has a considerable licence to remain ignorant of details which are

32

more comfortably left with the doctor. Of course, a good nurse knows as much as possible about her patient and her job which nowadays may involve the execution of complicated treatment and investigations. Nevertheless, the first purpose in nursing is to care for the sick and the nurse's professional image still tends to involve leaving all cleverness to other people. The ward sister may no longer be heard to snap, 'You are not paid to think, nurse!' (and any nurse trained 25 years ago knows just how common that was), but it is certainly true that the nurse is still paid (or rather underpaid — and physiotherapists are on much the same disgraceful pay scale) as a pair of hands and not as a magician. Nurses are expected to be paragons of kindness whereas doctors are expected to be paragons of cleverness. Physiotherapists are expected to be paragons of health itself — and to produce it as an emanation from trim figures and powerful fingertips. In practice, the physiotherapist is liable to be torn between her role as a highly trained independent therapist and her role as somebody who must blindly obey orders from the doctor.

Until this point, we have been looking at these matters in terms of the forces generally operating within hierarchies and between related professional groups; it is now necessary to examine the extra momentum resulting from sexual fantasies, sexual aspirations and sexual passions.

Chapter 3

The feminine professional image

Men are active in physiotherapy but they are a small minority. The typical physiotherapist tends to be pictured as a lithe young woman, good for a slap and tickle, or possibly a brawny lady with bulging biceps. One seminar member gloomily reminded us that, during the war, physiotherapists received the same extra rations as labourers; and they have to send their upper arm (biceps) circumference when ordering overalls. Physiotherapists are amused and exasperated but also fearful of these images.

More significant than the cardboard-figure silhouettes of the physio-therapist are the important real features of her self-image as a professional person. A crucial element is her use and misuse of feminity, her position as a woman who seems to be subservient to the doctor (inevitably pictured as a man — in the case of orthopaedic surgeons, he nearly always is). Complex reasons impel physiotherapists to adopt sometimes a caricature of passive feminity, akin to some of the bizarre gaits they are so good at imitating.

Firstly, people bring their upbringing and their own psychopathology to their professions and are liable to choose a profession on the basis of their own complicated predilections — even when it appears superficially to be a matter of accident and chance circumstance. Once in the profession, there are pressures to collude with the prevailing psychological configurations and defences. Idealisation of doctors may not be the main factor impelling a girl to become a physiotherapist but, once she has done so, she cannot avoid the tides of medical authority and magic that carry everyone in hospital. Any-one going into hospital for an operation wishes the surgeon to be something of a god and not merely the man next door; every person engaged in clinical work in the hospital shares these hopes and fears.

A number of the seminar members believed strongly that the central problem in the physiotherapy profession is its female domination. Their theory enshrined a degree of contempt for women that only a brave man or a fool would now declare in public. Since the seminar members were a group

34

who could command respect for themselves their self-contempt needs investigation. Apart from complaint about being in a women's profession kept down by men, they felt that physiotherapy has its own disastrous sexual features. The first complaint was that, as a professional group, they are incompetent bunglers with no leadership and no pride. They claimed that a male profession would have improved its technique and verified its efficacy long ago by a stringent scientific attitude, thorough, informed and infused with determined intellectual rigour. A male profession would be properly taught and trained, its methods tested, proven and applied instead of being amateurish, empirical and optimistic. Listening to all this, it was hard to realise that these are the same people who can describe a surgeon performing the fifth useless arthroplasty on some hapless patient, the same people who have learned to nurse the vanity of their medical bosses with consummate skill.

The situation, as caricatured, does correspond to current patterns and preconceptions. Social traditions mould educational habits and expectations and, in our society, there are rooted beliefs that girls are, or should be, less brainy than boys, possibly allowing, as compensation, that they should be more feeling, more sensitive, and better at intuitive guessing. Psychoanalysis, in seeking to contribute its theories and explanations for these patterns, sometimes appears to be reinforcing them. Better educational opportunity for boys is only partly explained by traditions of male privilege; there are also cogent, deeply-held beliefs — partly unconscious — about the nature of men and women, with which some of these social patterns conform. The stereotypes of intellectual men and emotional women are promoted by tradition and social expectation on conscious and unconscious levels and the two forces, external (society and tradition) and internal (the unconscious, fantasy life), are interdependent.

It seemed to me that the picture of the physiotherapy profession as a flock of twittering women contrasting with doctors as a race of sternly logical scientists belonged to the realms of fantasy and was not a real sociological proposition. The fantasy is of crucial importance. The unconscious beliefs underlying the work of the physiotherapist are confused and conflicting. They are fraught with confused ideas of bisexuality.

Owing to the nature of physical sexual differences and owing to the ubiquitous facts of childbirth and infant-rearing, certain psychological features tend to become regularly and differently associated with the two sexes. Feminine hopes and anxieties are more concerned with the interior of the body, its condition and products, and also with holding and containing. The male is more vested in the exterior and in performance and also in penetration (rather than containment). These different trends are comparative and formulated generally but they are, of course, not absolute or universal.

People with anxieties about the interior of the body often join the medical and paramedical professions and their choice of branch or specialty may reflect their personal defence configurations. Surgeon and physician are impelled by different ideals and different types of woe.

The physiotherapist must have special ideas and anxieties of her own. She will not have the narcissistic zeal of the actress or ballet dancer, but a certain pride in her body must be there as a professional hallmark. The balance of femininity and masculinity in that pride may be delicate, variable — and of key importance in determining the way she works and how she enjoys it. The preoccupation with mobility, muscular power and co-ordination is probably felt to be rather male, rather phallic in character. The use of 'apparatus' and gadgets would also tend to have the same type of unconscious significance. The yearning for scientific method and logic, as a firm supporting structure to thought, is also liable to be linked, unconsciously, with maleness, with the fantasy of the erect penis inside. For all of these reasons, the woman physiotherapist often feels herself to be striving in a man's world and with male aspirations, but without male equipment. This is what reinforces the feelings that 'a man would do this so much better'.

On the other hand, the capacity for patience, the staying power, the ability to observe, to hold and to care — all these aspects of the work will be in harmony with the common preconceptions of femininity. (It is re-emphasised that these remarks refer particularly to ubiquitous unconscious imagery, and are not offered here as a prescription for how people ought to shape themselves.)

Although it enrages physiotherapists to be described as 'good fairies' (and this evidently happens) who massage the male ego and preserve male illusions from bruising, they know that some of their fury stems from the grain of truth. They feel patronised by the epithet of 'good fairy' which could imply omnipotent powers of magic and kindness — and, a psychoanalyst might add, bisexuality. The dream-ideal physiotherapist is the perfect mother who holds you as long as you need it but never too long to let you mature — and she has the magician's powers to teach, in her magic wand, her omniscience and the omnipotence of her (phallic) apparatus.

Physiotherapists are serious professional women valued for imaginery powers they never claimed but are not respected properly as honest professionals. Their anger at this situation seems to come from disguised anxiety at the implicit confession of male weakness as much as from direct resentment of male scorn. Expectations of marvels from an ideal bisexual figure are easy enough to put into words and to understand, but they are very bewildering to the person who has to live up to them. Physiotherapists sometimes convey an intense sense of their bewilderment — the double-bind of being expected to be a soft cushion against reality and, simultaneously, to be resources of brain and thrust.

The posture of passivity, the feminine-caricature stance, is possibly a defensive reaction from the phallic aspects of their bisexual role. At the conscious level, the air of the delicate flower might be cultivated to offset fears of looking too brawny to be sexually appealing, and this could spill over into a pose as the dumb female to cover a degree of braininess that might frighten men. The anxious examination of the biceps circumference is a displacement from other parts of the body and from gender anxieties.

The foregoing has been concerned with the pressures on the physiotherapist to be omnipotent, not just in some vague general way but in a way linked intimately with her sexual identity. (This see-saws with the universal pressure to thrust the doctor into the role of God the Father and, with equal regularity, to chop him down again.) Her conflict about sexual identity, as underlying her therapeutic powers, reverberates with these tensions. She idealises the doctor because hope against death might be along that path — but she also idealises him to offset the guilt about her own unacceptable aspirations and as a reaction against the secret manliness she has been cultivating in herself.

If illness and death drive us to seek omnipotent figures and objects for our salvation, matters are greatly complicated by our primitive association of the processes of creation and death with the sexual nature of our parents and ourselves. The breast, the womb, the baby, the penis, the stool, the stream of urine — these are the wonders of the ancient infant world, the natural phenomena of our formative years — and of the timeless unconscious mind. If we still seek magic, we seek it in sexually invested organs and their excitability. Any conscious sexual frisson — pleasurable or frustrating — between patient, doctor and physiotherapist, is only the tip of the iceberg.

The chapter on the paramedical role examined the stance of passive subservience towards doctors. It is easy to see the stake in idealising the doctor to sustain optimisim; in using the bossy doctor to escape responsibility; in undermining the doctor to satisfy envy or cravings for revenge. All this is further animated by less obvious unconscious sexual impulses and fantasies. Of course colleagues in any organisation can generate sexual excitement and conflict in one another but the situation in hospital is especially complicated because medical work centres on the human body and its hazards. Meeting over diseased bodies, excessive anxieties about disease and death, together with other unpromising circumstances, all militate against the establishment of normal adult heterosexual pleasure. All parties are pushed back toward the derivatives of stifled infantile sexuality and the realms of part-object relationships.[1] Outside work

[1] Part-object relationship: psychoanalytic term referring to a relationship in which the body parts and products are endowed with separate existence and volition. Thus, the infant might imagine the breast or the stool, for example, to be independent loving or menacing figures in his life. The persistence of such fantasies would greatly disturb the relationship of a nurse and an incontinent patient — or a physiotherapist treating a woman whose breast is amputated for cancer.

(or perhaps in reaction from it) a doctor and physiotherapist may settle into a comfortable adult sexual relationship and even get married. In the context of work they are liable to be caught up in a tangle of positions bearing only a superficial and tortured resemblance to that of men and women in love. What we observe is something more reminiscent of the unhappy marriages that present themselves in the divorce courts — unstable affairs, always breaking up and always repeating themselves. There are periods of great mutual esteem and pleasure but there is a constant gravitation towards painful and persistent patterns of misunderstanding.

Often, leaving to have a baby seems to promise the perfect solution to all of these conflicts — an ideal achievement of creativity in which it may be hoped that sexual roles will be re-established in clear demarcation. Surprisingly, the women in the seminar never found it easy to believe that male doctors might actually envy them their feminine qualities and potentialities, even though they were so often in the role of the mother upon whom the family relies. So often, there was 'no treatment except physiotherapy' for the hopeless case.

Chapter 4

A remedial profession?

Healers and helpers. Community of purpose is economical and attractive and it succeeds if different professions can work together or in parallel, abandoning their trademarks. At times, there is little to distinguish the physiotherapist's work from the social worker's; and occasionally, the ward sister assumes the role of both. (Those cases where the physiotherapist is deeply involved in problems of discharging the patient from hospital illustrate the process, eg Cases 23, 27, 34 and 45.)

Because medical tasks do overlap, we are particularly concerned in the GP and Allied Professional Workshop to differentiate the various skills and impediments brought to the situation by each discipline. The biggest single surprise, to the author, in the course of the seminar with physiotherapists was the extent of their patients' chronic severe illness and extreme old age. In addition, physiotherapists have to perform their tasks encumbered by difficulties that do not exist in the same way for doctors and nurses. There is a more subtle and rather specific element in this situation that renders physiotherapists themselves unaware of their own predicament: they are supposed to be 'a remedial profession'. Doctors and nurses want their patients to make progress and to get better, but the doctor and nurse are licensed for their patients to get worse and die. By contrast, the physiotherapist is a 'remedial therapist' and does not have a respectable position around the deathbed. Yet she is often nearby.

Doctors and nurses have the task of remaining with patients in and out of illness, through disease and recovery, through the progress of disease and old age to death. A recognised part of their work is to ease patients through final illnesses, to nurse and palliate — and to accompany.

The physiotherapist is caught in a quite different position, forced to believe for as long as possible that she provides remedial treatment. A great part of the physiotherapist's function is indeed palliative and supportive: sustaining the diminishing physical resources of deteriorating patients,

39

and teaching them to do as much as possible with their remaining physical powers. Teaching a chair-bound paraplegic how to move from one seat to another, or how to get on and off the toilet with only one person to help rather than two — such achievements are momentous for the patient although far from the pictures of rippling muscles and strong fingers usually associated with physiotherapy. But physiotherapists cannot provide a remedy for the terminally ill.

Similar or even greater difficulty occurs with work which seems to be frankly futile and 'not physiotherapy at all'. Many patients are referred to physiotherapy departments because the doctor can't think of anything else to propose and although at first sight this seems to be quite wrong — one more instance of medical villiany — reflection makes the matter less certain. Psychoanalysts and psychiatrists are often concerned with notions of 'containment' and 'the holding environment' (our thinking on these matters owes much to W R Bion and D W Winnicott). In hospital life, the physiotherapy department can contain, hold and carry some incurable patients better than anyone else, although the physiotherapist may feel that it is a poor best. But since there is often no one to support or contain the physiotherapist, she has then to contain, within herself, a great deal of anguish, futility, humiliation and resentment.

A specific difficulty-cum-strength for physiotherapists with all their patients, but especially with these chronic patients, is the length of time they are together. This is central to the role of the physiotherapist as 'container'. Many procedures in physiotherapy require a fair amount of time — time rarely passed in silence. Unless she can develop perverse skills in not hearing and knowing, the physiotherapist is exposed to the patient's thoughts and anxieties. The doctor has the option whether or not to entangle himself in lengthy conversations with his patients but the physiotherapist does not have this choice.

Physiotherapists' training and expectations do not prepare them for prolonged work with the chronic sick, especially for lengthy tête-à-tête conversations. In fact, they are often taught not to involve themselves in discussions of the patient's condition and to refer such matters to the doctor. Time and personal aptitude may remedy these deficiencies but often they develop a range of tricks to abet them. Physiotherapists maintain elaborate routines to save time — some genuine, others not — in which they have several patients on the go at once and are constantly popping in and out of cubicles. They can do this with even one patient. At times, they seem to fear imprisonment with the patient and they slip out for cups of coffee or an early lunch, or go and switch things on and off; all this can make them increasingly tense, anxious or even quarrelsome. The underlying problem is the conflict between an overt purpose as remedial therapist and a covert purpose as supportive therapist, not only to the chronic sick but also to the professional colleagues for whom the physiotherapist is herself a crutch.

The material of the physiotherapist as crutch is an alloy of optimism. A degree of optimism is intrinsic to the work of physiotherapy and it is dangerous to confront this with too much honest doubt and scepticism, especially when the work is so often hopeless. In the long run it may be better to know than not, better to face reality than avoid it. Yet it does take time to shed the rigid and brittle defences upon which traditional medical and paramedical postures are often based. To interfere with optimism seems sometimes to interfere with the essence of physiotherapy. Whereas a bit of pessimism in the doctor may bring him much closer to his patient, pessimism in the physiotherapist is often incompatible with continuing the work in hand.

There are many double-binds.[1] Thus, the physiotherapist is required to be optimistic because her therapy demands it; she also realises that the case is hopeless because that excuses the colleagues who passed the case to her. She colludes with evasiveness and a systematic deafness to misery (the way hopeless illness is generally managed); she is also vigilant, observant and of sterling integrity (qualities fundamental to medical tradition). She takes the greatest professional pride in her work; she is also willing to be a humbug, a charlatan, and to agree that black is white if a doctor requires it. She relies on the doctor and defers to him because he knows best; but she often carries him like a baby when he is helpless and cannot clean up his own mess. These are some of the double-binds that generate bizarre behaviour in physiotherapists or lead to the response of leaving the profession.

Apart from the relief of pain, the great issue in the management of serious illness, with patients approaching death, is prognosis. When diagnosis and prognosis are discussed honestly, patients often require less analgesic drugs and sedatives. Pain feels much worse when it is compounded with fear, uncertainty and anger.

Patients all know that 'they never tell you anything' and hospital staff, on the other hand, complain of the way patients 'never take things in'. Between the two, a great many patients — perhaps the majority — reach their final days without explicit awareness of their fatal illness. This is common knowledge and common complaint. Some medical people remain convinced that matters are best left this way and there are, undoubtedly, some patients for whom this is the best way. A policy of telling, ensuring that the patient knows his position, has implications that require attention.

---

[1] Double-bind — the predicament created by simultaneous instructions or messages that are conflicting and incompatible. Some psychiatrists believe that mental illness may be predetermined by rearing in families where the child is constantly caught in a double-bind, whence insanity may appear to be a refuge. The most pathogenic double-binds in families are those that cannot easily be spotted. The same invisible processes go on in groups and organisations — and are rampant in hospitals.

Many management considerations involve quite banal decisions which can, nevertheless, be remarkably awkward. For instance, there must be some thought about the order in which people are informed — relatives first or patients first? And which person in the medical team does the telling? Beyond this lie the problems of support systems for the staff. In past times universal religious faith filled the present void. To read a 19th century novelist such as Charlotte Yonge is to realise that religion did not merely provide soothing answers for horrid questions: it also supported an ambiance in which discussion and explanation of anxieties about death freely occurred.

When patients are told the truth about their fatal illnesses, the staff have to meet the reactions and further questions. If patients are told that they are dying, the people caring for them will require mutual support to face the reactions, the complaints, the further questions, the disbelief and the human reality of the situation.

In the present state of medicine, the problem is somewhat different. The physiotherapist is nearly always situated in a network in which everybody is trying to avoid confronting the patient with the truth. The required support systems are now systems for secrecy and evasiveness. These systems impose enormous strains on hospital staff, much greater than the strains of a more honest climate. This contributes to the enormous drop-out rate from nursing and physiotherapy.

Losses from these professions are too easily attributed to poor pay and bad management. Pay is indeed disgracefully low, management is amateur and status is constantly undermined in all sorts of ways. However, illness and death are at the centre of professional difficulties in hospital and matters are worse in physiotherapy when the entire professional ethos places overwhelming value on cure and not care.

Physiotherapists are not careless or lacking in care but the notion of care carries the damp smell of death with it. Cure is a shining concept, clear and finite: care is a murky affair that belongs to the geriatric ward or, at best, the orphanage: it does not inspire the new recruit to physiotherapy, and it does not belong in the gymnasium. When cure is impossible, collusive secrecy and avoidance are the order of the day.

The physiotherapists' problem is similar to the problem for other hospital staff but, in certain respects, a degree more intense. More and more people in Britain now go to hospital to die but, in general, hospitals have not considered what to do with them. Hospitals are, very properly, factories in which to cure people: patients who are going to die are 'export rejects', 'seconds' or 'substandard'. The manufacturer whose imperfect goods are sold off in the January sales removes his trademark first and hospitals would dearly like to disclaim connection with their dead.

Cancer appeared during the second session of the seminar (8th March 1972) and the physiotherapist was struggling over whether 'to tell' the patient, although it was quite apparent that the patient already knew. Meanwhile, the physiotherapist performs mental acrobatics to remain not quite sure exactly what the doctor had said . . . This is one of the great areas in which physiotherapists hide behind the doctor's skirts. It is always possible to defer to authority in deciding when to speak out. Moreover, there is some substance in this. The physiotherapist will usually lack the overall view of the case that the doctor is supposed to have, but of course rarely does have in hospital. She knows that hers is a partial view and that she cannot responsibly speak out unless she accepts the further responsibility of knowing all about what is going on. It is always easier to leave it to the man supposedly at the helm.

Another case of cancer appears at the third meeting and, this time, the problem is neatly lost from two lucky chances. Firstly, the patient is deaf. Secondly, there is a most harmonious interdisciplinary team from which it does not emerge that any single person actually has the job of facing things with the patient. Hopefully, the social worker will be good at talking, although unfortunately, she does not know much more than a layman about breast cancer or the world of an operating theatre.

In the case of a fatal cerebral tumour (Case 36, 18th October, 1972) the patient's wife is admitted to a mental hospital while the medical team still collude with a man who entertains no doubt that he is going to make a 100 per cent recovery. In another case, described by the same physiotherapist (Case 61, 28th February, 1973) we see again how the conspiracy of secrecy about a cerebral tumour prevents the physiotherapist from establishing realistic priorities in the management and aims of treatment. In both cases, the patient is dead fairly soon and no one can be sure how much difference these issues made to him. But enormous burdens of anxiety and frustration were imposed upon the staff team at the hospital and on relatives. The drop-out from physiotherapy is, in part, the direct expression of such pressures.

For physiotherapists, even maternity leave takes on extra significance. Hospital staff suffer more than they realise from their proximity to disease and death and this gives an extra impetus, an extra dimension to the universal forces that lead people to think about procreation. The announcement of Ms Sycamore's pregnancy in the 47th session, 6th June, 1973, touched off complaints and envy about young women with better jobs. The really 'better job' in mind was maternity — and its 'betterness' was its antidote to professional anxieties, to gloomy impotence regarding incurable disease and ineffective treatments — as the remedy, in fact, for a distressed, remedial profession.

Physiotherapists are often near the deathbed, literally or psychologically but, in fact, suffer an important emotional deprivation in being excluded from a professional role at the moment of death. I recall only one instance in which we were told of the presence of a physiotherapist at the moment of death. To achieve this consummation, the physiotherapist was involved in a sudden death on an Underground railway station platform, and the session in which this was described was of unusual interest. The verbatim transcript of this session is discussed in Part III.

Death poses a multitude of problems and challenges for all who toil in the medical professions:

(a)   There are the problems of confronting or evading the emotions of the dying patient and those of his family before and after the death.

(b)   There are fears, humiliation and annihilation of omnipotent beliefs for oneself or one's idols.

(c)   And rarely admitted, there may be our own mourning problems.

The processes of mourning have been a central preoccupation of psycho-analysts ever since Abraham and Freud elaborated their thoughts on the subject around the time of the First World War. By mourning we mean those processes, involving some degree of misery, whereby a person comes to apprehend an important loss. The process consumes time and mental energy to work through the task of detachment and re-adjustment. According to psychoanalytic experience, mourning involves a variety of changing processes in the inner world of thought and fantasy life and, specifically, involves unconscious images of the lost object. A process of 'reality-testing' is involved whereby the bereaved person comes to apprehend and, in that sense, to accept the bereavement as a real fact. If these mourning processes are incomplete or if they are by-passed, the bereaved person may fail to make a stable adjustment to his loss and remains vulnerable to later vicissitudes that may reactivate them. Mourn-ing is, at depth, linked to early life's inevitable experiences of separation and disappointment. Psychoanalytic work indicates that earlier experi-ences of dependence and attachment, separation and detachment, involve anxieties and defences which may be closely akin to some of the anxieties and defences involved in bereavement and mourning.

On the whole, the problems of mourning are not widely supposed (ie noticed) to play a big part in the professional lives of doctors and nurses, let alone physiotherapists. This is because, in the main, we do not allow our patients to become, individually, figures of such importance to us that their death might constitute a grave personal loss. We may be more or less fond of our patients but, unless we have fallen badly out of role, we do not allow any one of them to become the light of our life. Never-theless, there are at least two sources of potential trouble.

First, some patients can indeed become very important to the person looking after them. Whether or not a departure from role is involved, there are many instances in the diary of the seminar where physiotherapists became entangled in an attachment to certain patients — though, of course, the attachment need not be one of unalloyed affection. Indeed it may be a relationship in which hostility and resentment predominant. Yet only a very naïve person would be surprised if the physiotherapists, in those instances, took it badly were the patient to die. It is common experience, as well as psychoanalytic theory, that pathological mourning is more likely to occur if a death is preceded by intense ambivalence rather than mutual love. 'Love 'em and leave 'em' has its validity at the deathbed as well as in child-rearing. If there is genuine and fulsome love, it is easier to separate, to allow the children to grow up and make their own lives: and the same love makes it possible to understand that a dead person has gone. Hospital personnel do become emotionally entangled with some patients and, thereby, become vulnerable to their deaths.

The second source of potential trouble is the entire class of factors that interfere with reality testing in the context of death. This includes the processes of idealisation, dissociation of awareness, addiction to omnipotent aspirations -- and kindred psychological defences. Much more obvious -- and so obvious as to be easily overlooked — is the concrete fact of not seeing the body. Of course it is not urged that every member of the medical team should see the body of every patient who dies. Unfortunately the physiotherapist almost never does, even though she has often been the person most concerned with the patient's body during life. The physical sight of a recently dead person is nearly always less ghastly than people imagine. Any actual ghastliness is likely to be a relic of mutilation during life rather than belonging to death itself. Disease and injury produce more horrid sights than death itself. (The question of viewing a body in advanced decomposition does not arise outside forensic contexts in this country.)

Funerals are for the living and are essential to initiate mourning processes and healthy engagement with the fact of a person's passing. The families of soldiers 'missing and presumed dead' in war have extraordinary difficulty in encompassing their predicament as long as it remains possible that the dead man is alive and going to come home again. Mothers of stillbirths have similar difficulties in adjusting to an unreal event, the death of a 'person' who never existed in ordinary reality -- and their difficulties are increased by the midwives' habit of whisking the stillbirth away, unseen.

For the physiotherapist, each fatally ill patient is liable to disappear, like a soldier reported missing and never seen again. Few physiotherapists would actually seek a role at the deathbed, but they would probably feel better if a legitimate role existed. This would do much to free them from the contradictions inherent in their role as a curing profession which has to treat the most incurable patients. Seeing the patient through to death would promote the grasp on reality that is otherwise eroded by the unreality of their 'remedial' ethos and by the disappearance of the dying patient. (Nowadays, physiotherapists are part of the team in intensive care units and this may have a useful side-effect since death must be more frequently seen in these units which are concerned with the most critically ill people.)

Chapter 5

Professional isolation

No man is an island. There is a basic human impulse to strive towards membership of a group, and, thence, towards group insularity. It sometimes seems that the consuming wish of a group is to function as an island, insulated from the world outside. Few men really wish to be islands by themselves, but a great deal of human endeavour (and romantic fiction) depends on the belief that a couple can, given luck, form a perfect island. Two's company and three's a crowd. Work in medicine and the allied professions involves a constant modulation between a state of existing in couples and a state of existing in groups, It is very easy to think of situations where one or other mode of existence is the more likely. The traditional family doctor is very often to be found in a one-to-one relationship with his patient, the hazard being that his independence of viewpoint may become submerged or lost in the entrancement a one-to-one relationship can afford. Of course this is not to imply anything unseemly or professionally improper, but rather to acknowledge the way a doctor can fail to realise when he is hooked by one patient — even if the relationship is one of quarrelling, or suspicion and exasperation.

On the other hand professional staff working in hospital derive great pleasure and support from a network of colleagues. The crowd will contain its assorted wallflowers and prima ballerinas but the majority function with some degree of integration in association with a group of colleagues. Some of the fashionable rose-tinted talk about hospital teams is remote from reality and, anyway, all groups and teams generate their own tensions. Nevertheless, hospital is, on the whole, a place for people who wish to work with others and not really the place for buccaneers and mavericks. Doctors have many different opportunities for sorting themselves out, from this point of view, and there is single-handed practice in the Hebrides for those who like to work on their own.

For physiotherapists it is more tricky. There are realms of private practice where they may work with considerable autonomy, solving most of their problems by themselves. We had only a glimpse of that sort of thing in this seminar, mainly when the physiotherapist was getting into difficulties. (For example, Case 5, 15th March, 1972; Case 44, 29th November, 1972 and various follow-ups thereafter.) It is worth noting that the price Ms Beech paid (Case 62, 28th February, 1973 to 28th March, 1973) for a confrontation with her superintendent was to be relegated to work in isolation in a remote part of the hospital. For that matter, it is also worth noting that Ms Beech was one of the very few members of the seminar who seemed to do much private work. It is probable that her personality turns her more readily in that direction and that isolation is less of a threat to her than to many others. By the same token, her arrangement with the seminar was sporadic and she left after two brief periods with us. A person of open and exuberant personality may still be something of a 'loner' at work.

Because of the tradition of working in a team in hospital, the physiotherapist may be all the more vulnerable if she becomes isolated. The difficulty is multiplied when this occurs covertly and she herself is not aware of it. It is quite possible to become seriously isolated from colleagues although working in conditions of positive overcrowding. For example, some patients have a knack of driving a wedge between colleagues and thus, in Case 4 (8th March, 1972), Ms Elm finds herself the only person standing between the patient and his fifth arthroplasty. The patient manages to play off the surgeon behind her back and is also able to mobilise a rather unpleasant rivalry between Ms Elm and her students. He gets his operation and is still haunting the out-patients clinic several months later. The same physiotherapist becomes isolated in quite a different way in Case 9 (28th March, 1972). This time she is somehow infected by the melancholy and isolation of the patient which has not been explicitly noticed and faced. She is occupied and possessed by her patient and, in consequence, loses awareness of the colleagues who could support her, such as medical colleagues in general practice or social workers outside the hospital. She feels, exactly like the patient, that she must carry everything herself.

A similar situation arises when the physiotherapist remains in prolonged contact with a chronic patient and therefore comes to have a unique importance for that patient. The hospital system permits and encourages a fragmentation of care and awareness. For most chronic patients, concern is disposed between several separate disciplines: doctors, nurses, physiotherapists, occupational therapists, laboratory staff, radiographers, social workers and others. Within each discipline, the problem is often further divided amongst a number of different people and more particularly, amongst a succession of different people, as the shifts change and staff come and go. The consultant in charge of the case sustains his own particular brand of continuity. His ultimate responsibility is one reason why he is paid a high salary; but the consultant is usually able to keep a safe distance, his visits are brief and his entourage is around him. Traditionally, the ward sister, in the same post for decades, did, and still does, carry a greater burden of continuous awareness of disease and its toll than anybody else in the hospital. This is now changing and the old picture may soon become part of a dying folklore as the organisation of the nursing team evolves into new configurations.

Quite often now, the physiotherapist is the one person who has been in close physical contact with the patient throughout a long illness and during many admissions to hospital. The situation is most likely to occur with a senior physiotherapist who does not frequently change jobs and does not leave to get married. However, personality type may count for more than age and two of our older seminar members were quite different in this respect. On the one hand, Ms Teak told us (Cases 55 and 56, 31st January, 1973) how much she preferred working with in-patients as compared with out-patients, because there was always a definite end to the treatment of in-patients. They would, at some point, inevitably be sent home and you were never saddled with them in the way that could occur with out-patients. (See, for example, Ms Poplar's Cases 20, 25, 26 and 39.) By contrast, Ms Oak reported a succession of instances in which she had come to occupy a special position for chronic in-patients. In Case 14, Ms Oak recognises what is going on and is successful in enabling the patient to detach herself — which means walking instead of remaining in a wheelchair! In Case 23, matters have become so distorted that the physiotherapist is landed with the job of arranging the patient's discharge until the seminar succeeded in disentangling her from this curious position. At a follow-up report (6th September, 1972), we hear that the medical social worker is reduced to tears by the problem, with Ms Oak providing cups of tea in the background. In Case 36, we again see the physiotherapist carrying rather more than her share of anguish about a case but, by contrast, we see in Case 43 that the same physiotherapist is quite capable of 'switching off'. She seems to have no recognition for a woman whose child she treated a few years ago — the child having now died.

Sometimes, it is the nature of the condition itself together with its treatment, that determines the special attachment of the physiotherapist to the case and, thence, her isolated detachment from her other hospital colleagues (ie non-physiotherapists). This happens in cases of severe arthritis and incurable paralysis of one kind and another where physiotherapy is the only treatment. In such cases the physiotherapist has a unique role in carrying the morale of her medical and nursing colleagues. She stands between them and the feelings that accompany complete helplessness.

Two factors combine at this point. *Firstly,* the severity and incurable character of the illness increase the likelihood that the patient will fall into the physiotherapist's lap. When the doctors can do nothing more, there is always the hope that physiotherapy may result in some slight alleviation and, failing that, the patient will at least be granted the illusion that something is being done. *Secondly*, the nature of the treatment throws the physiotherapist into intimate physical contact with the patient, for what may now amount to a life-sentence. No wonder that in the privacy of the seminar, we at times discussed the pros and cons of allowing a mother to murder her ill child, as if this really were an open question rather than an affront to all our avowed principles.

Sociologists and town-planners have long been aware of the problems of social isolation occurring in big cities, and one well-known problem is the vulnerability of the young mother living in a new housing estate where she doesn't know anybody, especially in a high-rise flat. The role of isolated mother can be crushingly difficult, generating depression or violence very easily, and it is very easy for medical personnel to find themselves in a similar position. The physiotherapist may feel that she is quite alone in carrying the burden of her patient's terrified, regressed infantile anxieties and demands. She herself is likely to feel murderous towards the dependant patient and towards her colleagues who have saddled her with the problem. The fact that, 'in reality', there may be no tenable grounds for grievance, makes it even more difficult to cope with her anger.

The physiotherapist is almost always surrounded by colleagues and often complains that it is impossible to get a bit of privacy with a patient. However, loss of privacy is by no means to be equated with the gain of companionship. The physiotherapist, surrounded by bustling colleagues, different echelons of her own and other hierarchies disappearing into the middle distance; the doctor existing in the background only as the person who firmly said, 'Over to you . . . ', all this can leave the physiotherapist and her patient marooned. There were cases where this process occurred in muted form but we also clearly felt that the physiotherapist consciously wished her favourite patient dead at times (Ms Oak's Case No 11; Ms Poplar's Case No 13).

The isolation process reached its most flagrant form in Ms Yew's Case No 74 (17th January, 1973). The mother of a congenitally quadriplegic child is preoccupied with the idea of murdering the child who is, in fact, safe in residential institutional care. The anxiety is transferred down the line and the young physiotherapist is persuaded to bring us the problem, in the seminar.

This case also illustrates a species of ambivalence which it is crucial for the professional care-giver to recognise. It is the dark side of the conspicuous and well-known love-hate that exists between mothers and babies or medical people and their patients. This is the conflict between admiration, on the one hand, and destructive envy on the other — all revolving around an idealised object in which hope is placed. In this case the seminar is confronted with a problem which is tormenting and impossible. The seminar and its leader are seen in the tricky idealised light of a psychological

Mecca. There is not only the hope that God can perform his celestial magic, but simultaneously the impulse to bring low and humiliate people rash enough to accept deification and pretend to perform the impossible. There is the perpetual hope that the therapist will possess wonderful powers — but she is also open to envious hatred if there is substance in the hope. Behind idealisation there always lurks the urge to humiliate. Thus the seminar is sent the case as a poisoned apple for the teacher. Physiotherapists, too, must beware of the flattering referral, 'I know you will be able to do something with this difficult case . . . ' By this point we have reached the antithesis of isolation and are in the suffocating regions where colleagues have become persecutors. Then it is a relief to be left alone.

Chapter 6

The case history: enough or too much

Taking the case history is the most important part of a medical examination — such is the gospel taught to every British medical student. Woe to the medical student who auscultates before he has palpated, palpated before he has looked, and doom if he does any of this before he has taken a good history. The new medical student wades through an interminable check-list of questions of whose possible relevance he has little understanding and often contrives to miss the crucial points. As his knowledge increases, his technique becomes more economical and by the time he passes his final examinations he has a reasonable nose for what is important — *medically speaking*. One of the most important skills he learns is how to parry the talkative patients, how to stop the flow of 'useless information' and extract the crucial pointers to the real nature of the trouble — *medically speaking*.

General practitioners are more in touch with their patients' lives and families than their hospital colleagues. General practitioners have, therefore, been quicker to discover (re-discover?) the messages to be heard if the ears are not plugged. A woman complaining of backache may be telling her doctor about compression of spinal nerves but she may be also stating that her husband's impotence gives her the hump. It is possible to remember the latter without forgetting the former.

Doctors — especially general practitioners — have long been confidants and advisers. There may be some division of interest between physical and psychological matters but attention to the psyche is inescapably part of their work. GPs know the necessity of this work — work for which they are rarely prepared in medical schools. They react in various ways. Some are resentful or even feel persecuted by the psychological demands of patients. Most succeed in teaching themselves and each other how to handle these demands. And a small percentage of zealots attend seminars to study these problems.

The position of the physiotherapist is very different from that of the doctor and much nearer to the position of the nurse. She has hardly any training or licence for history-taking, beyond establishing the bare physical data regarding a pain or injury. On the other hand, her contact with the patient is lengthy, or at any rate recurrent, and she has some licence to chat while she works, if the mood takes her. In consequence she is liable to pick up all sorts of charged information in the form of gossip. There is no agreed sense that the information might be useful nor any sanction as to how it may be used. A healthy inclination to test or verify details of the history is undermined by the lack of an overt sense that a history has legitimately been collected.

The doctor's case-history is intended primarily to help him towards a physical diagnosis. Its secondary functions are rarely proclaimed in the medical school. Sometimes, especially in general practice, secondary functions are secondary only in the sense that they are unavowed and in fact they may be the prime purpose. One such function is to provide time and space in which the doctor and patient can be together, establish rapport, build trust and get used to each other. Much of what goes on is akin to mating behaviour in birds where the establishment of a partnership is the primary event whatever the commotion. Another function of the overt history-taking — never admitted into consciousness and needing the collusion of doctor and patient — is to avoid hearing about the more disturbing covert case history. The proliferation and reiteration of detail about certain symptoms and certain events enables silence to be maintained about other things. Doctor and patient suppress the unpleasant truths. This process will inform the final physical diagnosis and will influence the chosen treatment.

Each doctor develops an unconscious art of history-taking which enables him to spend as much time as he can bear with the patient. This provides a sense of contact and familiarity as close as both parties can comfortably sustain while avoiding the emergence of information that would become a mutual liability, if brought into the open. Interference with this delicate balance is like interfering with many other of Nature's ecological arrangements and can carry unexpected results. For example, one GP seminar decided to take a closer look at the ordinary work of GPs by studying random cases. Each doctor would agree to report what he knew and what happened with the fifth patient in the surgery on Tuesday mornings.[1] One doctor's behaviour to the patient was so disturbed by this interference with his regular, safe habits that the patient felt able to press him for a loan of £50, a quite extraordinary event. The next week, the fifth 'random' patient

[1] We have now learned to randomise any such enquiry much more widely — not so much in the vain hope of scientific purity as simply to avoid gross and unproductive distortion of the doctor's work.

horrified the doctor by the unexpected disclosure of a saga of sexual perversions, the GP having known her as a staid, quietly married woman for over 20 years. The GP himself was so upset by all this that he left the seminar. An extreme case, but it serves to illustrate the nature of routine methods as a safety device not to be tampered with.

The physiotherapist knows about the importance of her case-histories but she is not *really* taught how to take them. Moreover, she rarely expects to take a history properly. In addition, she always seems to feel a charlatan when she is treating psychological illness or psychogenic symptoms and disabilities. Her options are much more restricted than those of the doctor, and the style of history-taking appropriate to the medical role cannot be altogether appropriate to the role of the physiotherapist.

To put the matter much more simply, she must devise a mode of enquiry that is appropriate to her problems with the patient and consonant with her opportunities. The impression provided by the seminar is that if they set about taking a history in a direct fashion physiotherapists find it difficult to escape from feeling uncomfortably like miniature orthopaedic surgeons or miniature psychiatrists. Many of them soon give up taking case histories altogether. Instead, they develop a technique for chatting with their patients and 'slipping in' questions on matters that interest them. A sizeable proportion of their patients suffer from psychological difficulties (even if there is a clear physical illness or injury too) and would like to ventilate them; but the climate of thought dictates an entirely physical approach.

This approach is built into the physical structure of nearly all physiotherapy departments where privacy appears to be almost unknown. Physiotherapists can use these physical conditions as an alibi for avoiding serious professional enquiry into the state of mind of their patients. Nearly all the members of the seminar emphasised the difficulty of finding anywhere quiet and private to talk to their patients, yet there is an enormous amount of information the physiotherapist can obtain and digest if she is so minded. On the other hand, it is fascinating to note the astounding agility in avoiding uncomfortable knowledge. Not only do these therapists often manage to avoid knowing much about their patients' lives but they also manage to avoid grasping the central medical facts of the case — the diagnosis and, above all, the prognosis. Time and again people would present cases where the prognosis must have been an overwhelming factor in determining the patient's state of mind and the appropriate treatment, yet the physiotherapist would have only a vague idea of the situation. The patient had undergone an operation for cancer but the therapist did not know whether the patient knew the diagnosis. Another condition might be crippling but the therapist wasn't quite sure of the nature of the illness or the prognosis. The seminar would often collude in an evasive discussion of such cases, avoiding the delicate and central issue. To ask would be tactless and it was often left to the seminar leader to spoil everybody's peace of mind by voicing the awkward question.

A frequent variation is for the physiotherapist to feel indignant about being left in the dark. The patient is referred with a garbled message or a small piece of paper with hardly anything on it. ('Backache – try traction'.) The patient quotes the doctor but the therapist does not know what the doctor actually said. In these aggrieved situations the physiotherapist was often unconsciously glad to shelter behind indignation while she remained ignorant of uncomfortable facts. It is easier to be able to tell the patient you don't know than to lie, dissimulate, evade or, indeed, to tell the truth when everyone about you wants to avoid it.

Sometimes, the sense of its-best-not-to-know hangs so thick in the air, possibly by diffusion from another case altogether, that even appropriate basic medical curiosity is extinguished. Doctors may lapse into extraordinary medical incompetence and blindness when their functioning and their state of mind is clouded by emotional disturbance – although this may be far from obvious. The anxiety may not be apparent in the conventional sense but may masquerade as casualness, impulsiveness, light-hearted forgetfulness and so on. Similarly, a physiotherapist may treat a patient for unusual multiple injuries after an accident but somehow manage to avoid finding out anything at all about how the accident occurred (Case 10, 28th March, 1972). It might be too disturbing to face a particularly painful instance of aged decrepitude, or the depression lying behind the negligent self-destructive behaviour that led to an accident.

Most medical personnel find considerable support from working in teams and, at its best, this means that different members of the team can do more for their patients and bear more anxiety than any of them could do separately. But every student of group behaviour knows that groups engender their own pathology and the team spirit may often be a brand of insanity. So often, the hospital team is concerted in its determination to prevent any of its members finding out what is going on. Information and the responsibility for it are fragmented and dispersed.

In one impressive instance (Case 23, 27th July, 1972; 6th September, 1972), they could not understand why it was so difficult to discharge a dear old lady into the arms of her devoted family. Ms Oak is a physiotherapist with a certain predilection for mothering people. This confused her team and she was landed with the job of arranging the discharge of this patient from hospital. Somehow, nothing was moving forward. The seminar showed Ms Oak that this was part of a collusion for everybody to escape the facts and avoid facing them in an appropriate way. Getting the physiotherapist to take over the arrangements was tantamount to ensuring that the facts of the domestic situation would not be systematically examined. After that, it was possible to delineate a difficult family situation. The medical social worker was restored to her correct role and slowly enabled to cope with it (Ms Oak's motherly propensities finding new expression in supporting the social worker).

Chapter 7

Anxieties and physical contact

It is curious that physiotherapists, who are in some ways closer to teachers than to any other profession, should be antipathetic to the notion that they are working in a field of psychology. True, a certain amount of their work is purely technical (the use of infra-red and ultra-sonic equipment for example), and much of their work is preoccupied with anatomical considerations; they may, with some reluctance (see page 61), perform massage or manipulation. The greatest part of their work, however, and the part that gives the most satisfaction, is teaching their patients to use their own faculties. Teachers know that they are working with other people's minds and, to that extent, physiotherapists must know this too: yet it is remarkable how they resent working with people who are not suffering from an organic physical disability. Case 19 provides an example of the way the physiotherapist can perform sensitive, useful work in this field, clarifying the diagnosis and assisting towards the evolution of the best management. Cases 25 and 29 show the way a physiotherapist can be torn apart by conflicting aims and loyalties in these cases.

Doctors and physiotherapists tend to feel deceived by patients with hysterical disabilities and the diagnosis then carries the aura of detecting a crime.

All sorts of difficulties proliferate when the situation cannot be frankly stated, when there is a facade in which nobody believes and when the physiotherapist feels mocked and exploited by the doctor or patient or both. Moreover, even when the doctor is perfectly frank about the nature of his referral and his sincere belief that the physiotherapist can successfully treat a patient with an hysterical disability, physiotherapists still feel bitterly resentful. The seminar repeatedly voiced the idea that their profession was used as a dustbin by doctors; that they felt themselves to be abused, belittled, and turned into charlatans. This was impressively shown in the very first session of the seminar. (Ms Oak's Case 2, 1st March, 1972)

57

when the physiotherapist was able to achieve an astonishing success in the case of a chronic hysterical disability of crippling extent. She achieved this in a matter of weeks whereas the doctor 'had been messing about in out-patients for a couple of years'. Nevertheless, the unanimous voice of the seminar was that of humiliation and exasperation. The physiotherapist may feel happily abandoned in her use of cajolement and pretence to encourage a patient with a physical disorder, but she finds it almost impossible to maintain self-respect when she pits her mind against the mind of a patient whose disorder is frankly psychological.

Psychological disorders and hysterical disabilities are upsetting to medical teams for many reasons: the sense of affront and deception, the exaspera-tion of staff devoted to curing physical illness when confronted with conditions that seem to be imaginary. Moreover, members of medical teams find themselves suddenly reduced from positions as skilled technicians to that of unskilled amateurs. These factors combine in the frequent 'explanation' of such cases as compensation neurosis or some similar state of affairs in which the patient is believed to be deliberately (or semi-consciously) pretend-ing to be disabled to achieve some rather obvious benefit. These explanations satisfy the therapist's injured feelings of being deceived as well as her deeply wounded professional humiliation at not really understanding the case at all.

Foolishness, born of aversion from unconscious anxiety, can overwhelm the cleverest of us. A High Court judge (no fool), sentencing a compulsive arsonist to a long prison sentence, declared his view that the worst aspect of the case was the fact that the accused had started all these fires in order to gain the few shillings he earned from overtime calls in the Fire Brigade. (His preoccupation with fires had, of course, been the real reason for joining the Fire Brigade.) In any other context, this would appear to be the credulity of an imbecile.

There are indeed *three profound factors*, all interconnected, that domin-ate these issues and hinder techniques suitable for coping with them:

1. Patient and therapist share an unconscious (or conscious!) awareness of the deeper meaning of much neurotic illness and hysteria, which tend to be rooted in sexual and aggressive urges. They feel unable to confront these urges and fantasies consciously and openly.

2. Bodily exposure and close physical contact in the treatment may carry an emotional charge which can rarely be openly recognised in the thera-peutic situation. Patients and those who treat them have to suppress sexual arousal or even any thought of it.

3. The psychiatrist's methods of work, based as they are on physical abstin-ence and distance, as a condition of maximal psychological expression, are totally irrelevant to the working ambience of the physiotherapist. But

his model distracts and overshadows — as if it were the only way of approaching emotional problems — and impedes the physiotherapist from developing the strength of her own position.

Sometimes, the element of sexual excitement as a disturbance is barely disguised and can even be viewed with a degree of good humour. In the case of Ms Elm's elderly lady (Case No 52) it is difficult to be angry with the son who wants Ms Elm to give him massage for his backache but this is the sort of episode that may be more comical to describe than to experience. What is less obvious is the sexual jealousy in the family, involving the therapist in tensions over secret glasses of whisky and secret cups of tea, in tense conspiratorial circumstances. Ms Elm is angrily aware that, in being pushed into giving the old lady a bath, she is caught up in forces that she can only dimly understand. She would not recognise them as sexual and, neither perhaps may some readers. There is probably a vicious circle in this type of situation. Sexual thrills (overt or disguised) are a prime defence against anxiety about health and life, but they carry their own aftermath of guilt and further anxiety. The son who wants Ms Elm to massage his back is not simply expressing *joie de vivre*; he is not simply out to sample the pleasure any healthy young man might seek with an attractive young woman. He does not, to put matters in basic terms, invite Ms Elm out to dinner or into bed. What he does is to state his unconscious theory that sexually-tinged attention is the required cure for anxiety and illness: hence the request, quite logically, for her to treat his backache. We may also guess that the sexual attentions and thrills have an infantile character to them — we sense the mixture of childish appeal and sexual provocation in his request. We are also able to recognise the same elements in the behaviour of the elderly mother who gets Ms Elm to bath her. It is easy to understand that the members of this family are pitched about by their jealous passions involving one another and by the guilt and fear generated.

In Case 50, the initial suspicion that this was a case of compensation neurosis gives way to the awareness that the patient has matrimonial difficulties and that he wants the physiotherapist to provide disguised sexual gratification. ('He really wants a floozie.') Unresolved conflict in these anxious areas may be a frequent reason for patients otherwise inexplicably breaking off treatment, as occurred in this particular case.

It is common knowledge that some embarrassing problems may more easily be discussed with a total stranger than with somebody you know. The family doctor is often a more suitable confidante than a member of one's own family but sometimes patients will say that even he is too familiar, too close, and they may prefer to take their problems to the anonymity of the hospital. Each clinician (doctor, social worker, nurse or physiotherapist) has to strike the right balance between amiable familiarity and cold distance. The issue is enormously affected by the element of physical contact. Generally, embarrassment is thought to be minimised by the greatest dissociation of physical intimacy from talk and inter-personal recognition. Intimate physical examinations tend to be performed in silence or accompanied by the exchange of innocent and neutral banalities: any conversation continues afterwards as if nothing had happened. Indeed, the white coat and the clinical demeanour enable essential physical examinations to be carried out without fuss. Medical evangelism has overcome religious and social taboos. We have thereby developed other taboos, especially against interpersonal awareness. It may be impossible to achieve intimate physical access and intimate psychological access at the same time, in clinical work.

In general, it works reasonably well — those who minister to the patient's body do not have too much to do with his psychological problems and conversely, those who struggle with the psyche avoid the laying on of hands.

A rigid psychoanalytic tradition has evolved, whereby psychoanalysts eschew completely any other role as medical attendant to their patients and bar themselves from all physical contact, beyond an occasional handshake. Indeed, most psychoanalysts work within a technique of studied neutrality and distance from their patients. This psychoanalytic technique is akin to the white coat and businesslike manner of the gynaecologist and the aseptic technique of the surgeon. It is not a blueprint for all therapists grappling with psychological problems in different patients and in other situations.

Freud had some hard lessons to learn before his later techniques evolved; and problems of erotic emotional transference caused violent disturbance in the early history of psychoanalysis. It is still startling to read, in one of his very earliest papers, of his treatment of one Viennese lady. Not only were there daily sessions of abreaction under hypnosis but, ' . . . I massaged her whole body twice a day'. Psychoanalysis or physiotherapy?[1]

The dissociation of personal intimacy from medical physical intimacies remains the most comfortable arrangement so far as the majority of people are concerned. We had, therefore, to work hard in the seminar to reinstate a sense of the possibilities for psychological (as distinct from psychiatric) work within the *modus operandi* of the physiotherapist. But the psychiatric interview is not the only model that may be employed for talking with patients: the physiotherapist can learn to use the power of her physical intimacy with the patient, where a few words go a long way. There is no room for over-simplicity or rules of thumb in such matters. Some patients will feel far too insecure to talk without their clothes on, feeling that their self-control is a precarious affair and that their impulses are already too near

---

[1] 'The Case of Frau Emmy von N', in *Studies on Hysteria* (1895), Sigmund Freud, Standard Edition, Vol. 2, Hogarth Press and Institute of Psychoanalysis.

the surface. The physiotherapist may be able to build a sense of the person she is dealing with *by noticing* which way the pendulum swings, emotionally, as there are more or fewer clothes on.

To notice these things does require a dislocation of the physiotherapist from much of her former training and from traditional attitudes. Doctors, nurses and the rest of us working in medicine learn very early to grow a shell of seeming impervious to embarrassment or even, sometimes, to awareness of which parts of our patients' bodies are showing. The proctologist lives his life in the rectum with as little or as much excitement as a window cleaner. But the window cleaner has the advantage and there is no serious impropriety in George Formby singing saucy songs about it all whereas there is not much toleration for anybody who has a giggle about what the doctor or the nurse saw. Here is another dilemma, another double-bind. If the doctor, the nurse and the physiotherapist stayed consciously aware of all the frissons of sexual excitement, infantile anxiety and glee as they approached the patient's body, they would most likely be unable to carry on their work for very long without a nervous breakdown. On the other hand, the dissociation, coldness and impartiality that are assumed prevent them from understanding their patients and learning what they are trying to convey. Moreover, medical people feel invaded and angry when certain patients somehow do manage to get through these defences. It is no derogation of the technical skill of physiotherapists to speakof the enormous psychological component in their work — yet such remarks do touch a very sore spot. The soreness may have much more to do with the unconscious nature of hysteria than with the technical and professional status of physiotherapy. Awareness, knowledge (even at the unconscious level) of what the hysteric is up to and how his bodily parts are invested with erotic and aggressive fantasy, is embarrassing and profoundly disturbing to someone who must nevertheless go on handling them.

Aspects of massage

Massage is out of fashion and, in some circles, a dirty word. Freud might almost be said to have discovered psychoanalysis during his treatment of Frau Emmy von N, with sessions of hypnosis and massage to the entire body twice daily. Since then, with the growth of psychological awareness about the unconscious impact of medical procedures and more sophisticated self-awareness within the healing professions, forms of treatment which openly include 'suggestion' and gratification of the patient by the doctor or therapist have declined. The spirit of the times now makes it quite hard for doctors to prescribe the assortment of bitter-sweet medicines that used to be so helpful to their patients and to themselves. We all used to enjoy a gullibility that is now outmoded as a more puritan spirit has taken over the professions. This may be a corollary of the spread of permissiveness and licence elsewhere.

People generally have much more freedom nowadays to sample the thrills and pleasures of sex, nudity, physical contact and open talk and this may have reduced the pressure on the medical and paramedical professions to provide the veiled forms of gratification and titillation, formerly in great demand from them.

It may be simply that old disguises have worn thin and transparent: new ones are necessary. The harmless bottle of coloured water on the mantelpiece has had to give place to the box of poisonous capsules in the bathroom cupboard. Doctors now have to be ready to discuss sexual intimacies with their patients whereas formerly the patient was gratified or fobbed off (whichever way you look at it) by physical examination and contact. The proliferation of elaborate medical investigations is not only a by-product of scientific advance: it is also a move away from intimacy and the more earthy modes of past doctoring. The 'examination from top to toe' is replaced by the chest X-ray and full blood count. Even the routine WR,[1] and its implications of adult-life-lived, is dying out.

Massage is out of fashion amongst physiotherapists and was mentioned very little in the seminar. These physiotherapists gave the impression that they hardly ever performed it and there were some indications that, if they were to decide on a course of massage for a patient, it might cause a commotion in the department and encounter a number of obstacles. The feeling was that massage is something for a sauna bath and Soho, not for a self-respecting paramedical profession. In the event, such robust reactions would probably be rationalised as an objection on grounds of time. There is a lot of resistance to the physiotherapist having a one-to-one relationship with any of her patients. The traditions are for her to keep several people on the go at once, settled in different corners and cubicles attached to apparatus or performing their exercises. A physiotherapist massaging somebody is totally monopolised by that patient for the duration of the treatment, and the time and mental energy taken up could extend quite a long way on either side of the actual period of massage.

The trend is away from intimate personal contact at a leisurely pace, towards impersonal, mechanical nontouch treatments — and hurry. Many of the desirable physical effects of massage may be achieved more easily with apparatus emanating comforting radiations. Massage may be very nice but infra-red is, we hope, just as good or even better — certainly quicker and cheaper. Yet, it is the difference between mother's arms and breast on the one side, compared with incubator and bottle on the other; and there are times when incubator and bottle are better or even life-saving.

Massage techniques (delivered by either sex) must often carry the unconscious significance of something akin to a basic or primary experience of mothering, since holding and comforting in intimate bodily contact are

[1] Wassermann Reaction: a blood test for syphilis.

central aspects of the mother-baby relationship. Whatever the social pressures and psychological meanings there is a move away from the physiotherapist-as-masseuse, the mother comforting the baby, towards the physiotherapist as a technician operating powerful contraptions and knobs. There has been a move from a maternal, feminine image to a phallic one. The second image, although phallic, is not a simple male or paternal one — it incorporates the sexual and magic features of both parents, as if some kind of partnership is embodied in one person. [Cf. ubiquitous bi-sexual images in nursery tales — the fairy with magic wand, the witch with cat and broomstick.] This is a very important variation or counter-part of the magic invested in doctors. In session 40, reprinted verbatim in Part 3, there is a close juxtaposition of irrational expections from gadgets (apparatus in Case 66, the ICD machine in Case 62) and an astonishing idealisation of surgeons.

Overdetermination[1] is involved at this point. It concerns yet a further factor that was neglected in our discussion in the 40th session, although ventilated occasionally during other sessions: the disgust and revulsion associated with touching.

Pursuing the maternal model, we should remember that the loving mother-baby couple are not merely erotic objects to each other. If massage were only a question of evoking forgotten delights at the breast and kindred pleasures that belong to other times and places there would merely be the problems of guilt relating to forbidden erotica. In real life the baby may be a disgusting and infuriating person and the mother has to overcome a tumult of difficult reactions in herself and in the child. While massage may sometimes be disturbed by guilt at the pleasure it affords, touching and feeling may also trigger different and powerful fantasies with reactions of fear and disgust. A physiotherapist who was feeling a patient's lump when it burst, spraying her with pus, was put off touching anybody else for quite a time. In the episode (Case 66) of the sudden death on the tube station, subsequent discussion suggests that we failed to recognise the problem of disgust, nausea at mouth-to-mouth breathing complicating the case. Ms Poplar remarked at the time on the association of other disgusting sights encountered in their work (eg suppurating wounds and bedsores) but mostly the reactions of disgust are well-covered by professional armour.

The lay public tends to overestimate the extent to which medical people are hardened by familiarity to gruesome sights. A degree of frequent daily exposure to mutilation of the body does produce a corresponding degree of

---

[1] Overdetermination: a term coined by Freud and Breuer in *Studies on Hysteria* (1895) and later developed extensively. It refers to the process where by a single item of behaviour or dreaming or psychopathology enshrines several different unconscious distur-bances and repressed wishes. It is a psychological version of killing two birds with one stone.

tolerance. One 'gets used to it'. However, in these days of wonder drugs and miracle surgery, it is possible to go through a medical training without seeing some of the gory sights that used to be common hospital experience. The writer was once doing a temporary job as an orthopaedic house surgeon and assisting at a rather nasty operation on an adolescent girl's knee. He was mildly surprised to be overtaken by faintness in the middle of the operation and had to be taken out of the operating theatre, to recover ignominiously in the corridor. What was more astonishing was to be joined a minute or two later by the experienced surgical registrar in a similar condition, led out by a nurse at each elbow.

'Getting used to it' is supposed to develop a thick skin which can be as thin as paper. The work of the seminar served to erode the defences of members, so that some did report the unexpected recrudescence of forgotten inhibitions and revulsion. Some seminar members became quite self-conscious about touching their patients or their colleagues, wondering if their students noticed their renewed anxieties. Possibly, the seminar did not do enough work on this front, but when we did get around to it, towards the end of our time together, quite a lot came out in a rush.

Relaxation techniques

From the physical point of view massage and relaxation approach various similar goals by rather different methods. From the psychological point of view, there are also differences — and the seminar helps us little as we never did these subjects full justice during the time we had — but there are also important similarities in the two approaches. Massage techniques and relaxation techniques both involve a heightened awareness of the body. In massage, this awareness is communicated wordlessly by close physical contact, whereas relaxation techniques depend on training the patient, from a distance, to develop a conscious and explicit awareness of bodily parts and so master the tensions that can control sensations and functioning.

Relaxation techniques in ante-natal training have swept the world, if not with all the success sometimes claimed. This is an area involving much idiosyncracy and variation from hospital to hospital. Often, the physio-therapist is confined to a restricted position of teaching exercises for breathing and exercises for the pelvic floor but not much else, whilst doctors, midwives and nurses all struggle along independently of one another, in a tower of Babel. Most people in the field recognise that although ante-natal classes may primarily be for training in certain exercises and in relaxation techniques, they also have an important function in providing the opportunity for expectant mothers to voice their anxieties and fantasies about their bodies and about forthcoming events. There are vast differences between different hospitals in the role of the physiotherapist in this situation. Sometimes, she is welcomed as a sophisticated counsellor and confidante, whereas in other places she may be forbidden to discuss anything except the weather lest she mislead a patient on some serious matter.

Retreat from physical contact

In summary, we see a retreat from the former popularity of massage and an inhibition from physical contact for several reasons. Firstly, some alternatives employing apparatus are quicker, convenient and efficacious. Secondly, the possibility of stimulating erotic feelings and fantasies in patient or therapist generates anxiety, leading to an embargo. Thirdly, there is the move from being the hum-drum comforting mother towards a world of man-made knobs and gadgets to which exaggerated healing powers are attributed. Fourthly, disgust and revulsion reinforce any tendency to physical withdrawal. Conversely, relaxation techniques can develop mutual awareness of the body with fewer problems of direct contact. Attentive mimicry is less noticed as an important method or expression of closeness without touching.

Chapter 8

Mimicry and trickery

Using mimicry

Demonstration and mimicry are vital items in the technical equipment of the physiotherapist teaching relaxation or exercises. I was struck by the extraordinary flair the physiotherapists seemed to develop for imitating their patients. It often seemed simpler for them to leave their chairs to demonstrate bizarre movements and paralytic gaits than to talk about them. The knack of imitating and simulating complex movements is a valuable resource for the physiotherapist struggling to convey instructions to patients who are not able to take in mere words. Physiotherapists are trained to analyse the components of complex movements and it follows logically that they should be able to pin down and copy a bizarre action or a peculiar gait that is bewildering to someone not so trained. However, the process extends beyond the mere intellectual application of anatomical knowledge. At times, the work with patients involving the closest attention and mutual copying also involves a special kind of bodily empathy. Many types of unconscious impulse and fantasy are involved in the conscious activities of imitation – fantasies, variously, of possession, occupation (as in preoccupation, being-occupied-by), and thence, ideas of invasion, control, etc. To see two people deeply involved in watching and copying each other is to realise just how immersed in each other they may be and, at times, how much the certainty of who is who is eroded.

Physiotherapy involves a closeness and intimacy which can be independent of physical contact or exposure and totally independent of psychological confidences. The particular type of attention the physiotherapist must sometimes bring to the way a patient's body behaves can involve a degree of unconscious identity-blurring. The professional skill of physical mimicry can even be carried over into a knack of imitating voices and thinking. A young lady with the King's English, consciously imitating a disgruntled old docker from Wapping, may be good-humouredly coping with a problem — but she may also be struggling with difficulties in distancing herself, at times seeming almost to become the docker.

Using trickery

The seminar sometimes gave the impression that physiotherapists are more often concerned with trickery than either nurses or doctors, except perhaps for neurologists. There is a fine line between tricks and trickery and cheating. Everybody enjoys a good conjuror because it satisfies primitive needs and anxieties. Life experience, from Day One, is a constant reminder that we hang by a thread, that the balance of forces far beyond our control is essential for our survival, and that things can be far more easily smashed than they can ever be put together again. If we do not all quite need gods, we certainly need magicians; and the prime minister who can pull something out of the hat is certain of a big majority in the next election. Unfortunately, trickery can become an addictive bad habit.

Physiotherapists use tricks all the time to find out what their patients can and cannot do in the way of movement, eg Case 5 discussed on 5th March, 1972, and they use tricks to enable patients to do things they were incapable of doing before. A spastic child being trained to walk will agree to push a trolley, although feeling unable to make steps otherwise. He can be tricked into using his hands to play a game although the same movements might not be forthcoming on direct request.

Similar techniques are in constant ingenious use in the physiotherapy department and are associated with dangerous undercurrents. To involve adults in games and tricks must mean, at some level, involving them in a degree of belittlement, tinged with mockery and contempt. This may be a small price to pay for success in getting a paralysed man to leave his wheelchair but some of the cases we discussed suggest that when matters do not go well, the tricks may have made things even worse. For some patients — and it is hard to know which in advance — dishonesty and condescension have the most deplorable effect. It is particularly necessary to be straightforward with patients who have already felt themselves to be tricked or let down.

In many of these cases, the physiotherapist meets the repercussions of somebody else's mismanagement or the patient's bad luck. It is with these patients that the physiotherapist is tempted to drum up hollow optimism and employ every tricky device at her disposal to gain a success. The patient's need to feel more genuinely supported may find expression in undue demandingness or anxious, suspicious mistrust, for example, in Case 21 (20th July, 1972) the case of the girl who awoke from the anaesthetic to find that her patella had been removed. Thereafter, she seemed unable to *trust* the strength of her own quadriceps muscles, or the reliability of the physiotherapist who was forced to keep holding her leg up for her. The girl had recently suffered the death of her mother and this underlines the problem for the therapist who had to be something like a reliable parent who supports a child. The problem involves being able to accept a degree of idealisation, or even to live up to it, without becoming (or feeling) a confidence trickster. Colleagues in hospitals can provide a vital amalgam, supporting one another in optimistic idealisation yet keeping within acceptable limits of reality and honesty.

The physiotherapist lacks a proper tradition, licence and habit regarding history-taking. As a result, this area of work is especially likely to be contaminated by trickiness. Instead of honest enquiry (which can still be tactful) there is the tendency to chat, slip in sly questions and pick up what you can. The difficulty is magnified when the area of enquiry is delicate and, above all, when the patient is suspected of malingering or of having produced a self-inflicted injury. This appears in the case of the man with the ulnar nerve injury — Case 30 (27th September, 1972). Some larger issues around history-taking have been discussed previously.

Sometimes, the staff slide into trickery when they feel hostile towards a patient. For example, in Ms Mahogany's Case 45 (27th September, 1972, 13th December, 1972) the man with severe rheumatoid arthritis. Is it simply that the staff are angry with a truly unpleasant man or are they struggling with the guilt and anxiety that his disability arouses in them, unconsciously? He is eventually discharged from hospital only by a trick. He is taken on a 'home visit' but the escort is told not to bring him back — the combined resources of a famous London hospital can be pushed or drawn into such contortions.

Trickery can also spring directly from staff difficulties rather than from anything specific about the particular patient. This is displayed in the report (6th September, 1972 — Ms Poplar) when appropriate discussion and management is completely submerged in the mystery-mongering, generated by staff anxieties, about the impending closure of the hospital. On the other hand, an extremely baffling and provocative patient (Ms Elm, Case 24, 27th July, 1972) brings out the worst in the hospital. The 'treatment' is a mixture of pretence, tricks and empirical trying-out: Ms Elm feels a charlatan and the patient knows it. She is cast in this role by the way the patient has been referred by the doctor, but there is an uneasy sense that the cap fits. Anyone treating this odd man feels helpless but, since hospital staff have no licence to feel helpless, they must pretend.

Trickery inevitably becomes entangled with deception and self-deception. The physiotherapist who tricks her patient, also deceives herself into believing that the patient has not found her out. The patient, at depth, always knows he has been tricked and the real problem is not whether he knows but, rather, how he is going to react.

Chapter 9

Transcript of a seminar session

This section contains the verbatim transcript of one meeting of the seminar. It is presented here for several reasons. Firstly, it conveys a sense of what the work of the seminar was like. In some important respects this session was atypical but it does show the seminar at work, struggling with unexpected difficulties and expressing, with particular frankness and clarity, quite a wide range of the anxieties and attitudes that prevail amongst physiotherapists. Secondly, the session is presented because it was a moving and somewhat crucial experience for us and highlights some of the central preoccupations of this book. Thirdly, it is reprinted now because it was a session previously transcribed and discussed in the GP and Allied Professional Workshop. This means that there is the opportunity to draw from the ideas and reactions of other seminar leaders who studied this transcript.

The session was atypical and was presented to the Workshop for discussion of certain technical problems which it posed for the seminar leader and which, in various guises, often occur in seminars. I was particularly interested in some discussion of the problems raised by unexpected material. It is the responsibility of the leader of the seminar to look after its boundaries and this does mean, at times, being an umpire who decides what is or is not admissible.

The problem occurs twice with little warning in this session. The first instance is Ms Poplar's — a case which may break the bounds of the seminar's work, if, as a number of people felt, it is not really an instance of the professional work of the physiotherapist but rather something that happened in her personal life, albeit on the way to work. The opposing view would be that this episode is a legitimate expression of the larger problem of how unmanageable personal experience can break into our professional work. We all have to recognise that, at times, our judgement and competence are enormously impaired (or occasionally heightened) by personal anxieties and preoccupations that arise from our private lives and personal make-up. It can therefore be argued that Ms Poplar's experience on Euston station was an episode on that tricky borderland between professional life and private life and that it was right for the seminar to struggle with it. We had already learned, in one of the opening sessions, that Ms Poplar has a sister who has a tumour with a bad prognosis, although we understood her to be in good health at that moment. She is tearful frequently during this material and we have to consider whether this is the common reaction of any sensitive person caught on the wrong foot, rather than an outlet for a great deal of pent-up emotion and anxiety. If so, are these pent-up emotions to be seen primarily as Ms Poplar's own affair or is this her version of problems that are really ubiquitous — in the seminar, if not throughout the profession.

The second wave of the unexpected is Ms Oak's case. Right at the beginning of the session, she mentions that she has a small addition or amendment to report from the previous week. This seemed reasonable to invite for the last 15 minutes of the session — to keep us up to date with other work and to get us back to earth. However, before the seminar leader realises what is happening, we are waist-deep in the complexities of a quite different case. The promised follow-up from the previous week comes only as an afterthought, in the last 60 seconds, whilst meantime the seminar is unexpectedly overwhelmed with a totally different problem of considerable complexity and difficulty. There is obviously something fishy about such a turn of events. As we listen, it is very difficult to know whether we may safely relax and admire Ms Oak's impressive clinical ability — a really extraordinary psychological touch, concealed under a superficial impression of rambling shapelessness. Her understanding of the case develops at astonishing speed and she moves it successfully towards a well-managed and appropriate psychiatric referral. However, she evidently suffers a considerable degree of tumult within herself as she does all this and her skill is mainly intuitive: she is neither supported nor impeded by a clear idea of what she is doing. We are left wondering whether the seminar should aim to make her less muddled, more self-aware and, maybe, less effective.

A preliminary word about the very first case today is also required. This is Case 62 and is its second follow-up. The original problem was a difficult woman with a facial palsy. She was referred, incredibly, for daily electrical stimulation but given no sense of the prognosis — which is fair but uncertain. The physiotherapist was, as usual, left uncertain exactly what the doctor may have said, humiliated and enraged at having to give a treatment which she felt to be useless — and at having to fob off an incredulous patient. The first report of the case centred around the collusion of the women involved, to maintain the doctor as an unseen idiot or bogey-man. The first follow-up described the tremendous row that ensued when Ms Beech had it out with her superintendent that they could not continue like that. There appeared to be an inpenetrable barrier

70

of superintendent, nurses, receptionists, secretary, all preventing access to the Great Man himself. As a result, it was established that she should 'do' one of his clinics with him to establish contact; and the other physiotherapists in the department were allocated a regular time each week to see him about problems, seemingly an excellent and most impressive development; but Ms Beech herself is simultaneously re-allocated to an isolated sphere of work on her own, in a remote part of the hospital, for the rest of the week. Today's follow-up describes the actual meeting with the Great Man himself. None of us realised, at the time, the degree of strain all this had imposed upon Ms Beech. Indeed, there was a feeling of optimism about the development that appeared to have been achieved in the department and within her own personality but it is now a matter of grim interest to go over the transcript with an eye open for the various points at which, with hindsight, it is possible to recognise the warnings emanating from her. We were quite amazed, at the time, when she disappeared from all subsequent meetings since the predominant impression had been of (for once!) very clear achievement and benefit.

Could we — or should we — have been able to spot her distress, concealed behind the successful development of her case and behind the much more obvious distress of Ms Poplar, in this session? When we all met again, 18 months later, Ms Beech described how she had felt the seminar (and especially its leader) to have failed to respond to Ms Poplar in a warm human fashion. She perceived Ms Poplar as having rashly trusted us with her inner feelings, only to be left isolated, the subject of cold academic curiosity. 'I decided that if I got my knickers in a twist I wouldn't come and tell you lot!' She left the seminar and took a long time to digest the whole experience. In retrospect, she thinks that there were elements of mismanagement and misunderstanding which contributed towards her sense of a cold-blooded dissection of human distress, in order for someone at the Tavistock to write a book.

A few other seminar leaders, contemplating the transcript, were inclined to agree with Ms Beech. Some agreed that the correct response of the leader (to Ms Poplar's case) should have been to accept — with the seminar members — that a very nasty thing had happened on the way to work: Ms Poplar *had* to talk to somebody and we should have accepted the role of sympathetic friends instead of trying to be clever.

Others felt the actual handling to have been justified and rewarding. Looking through the transcript, many important matters were able to come out, be noticed and discussed — issues that were intermittently perceived before but rarely with this clarity. It was also argued that Ms Poplar is probably not short of friends to tell her troubles to, if that were all she wanted: the seminar *should* be able to supply a type of attention and comprehension that would not be available elsewhere; we *should* rise to the occasion and not 'go humble', turning ourselves from professional colleagues into mere friendly neighbours. Arguably, that kind of warm 'human' response could really be a rejection and betrayal of trust, shirking the seminar's responsibility to provide serious professional attention, even if it hurts. Nobody would, after all, admire or condone a doctor who sent the patient home with friendly sympathy when careful but painful treatment might have ameliorated the condition presented.

This transcript has undergone minimal editing in order to remove a couple of passages it was considered inappropriate to include. The sense and balance of the session is retained in all essential respects.

The author's retrospective comments are interposed in brackets.

Transcript of a seminar session: Wednesday, 28th March, 1973

Poplar   Well I am sorry to say that I left a patient with somebody else and I came here *expressly* to talk, because I feel awful and I have got to talk. So there you are, that's one case.
(Somebody laughs)

Bourne   Right . . . does anybody else?

Oak   I have something to say, no, a correction to make . . . a supplement to last week.

(Note this remark, which completely misleads the seminar leader when we come to the last 15 minutes.)

Beech   I would just like to finish off that saga of mine. The facial palsy. It's just that I met the doctor and the doctor is a most reasonable man, an innovator and really great.
(Laughter)

Beech   His protection racket is unbelievable!
(Laughter)

Beech   That's really all there is to be said.

Bourne   Can you elaborate slightly, just for a couple of minutes, to clarify?

Beech   Well I did his clinic, I was allowed to do his clinic and he is a great guy. He's young, he's very much an innovator, his attitude to physios is excellent, the rapport was great from the word go and he discussed patients. He asked. You know, as he was diagnosing, he asked me what I thought. It was all you would want, but the protection outside until you actually get into the room to see him was just unbelievable. There is nothing really much more to say.

Oak   Who was guarding him?

Beech   Superintendent and assistant superintendent.

Sycamore   His secretary too because you indicated you had some trouble.

Beech   Yes, his secretary.

Mahogany   Well, they always do, don't they?

72

Beech	But, as a man he, he . . . I don't think he is *aware* that it's going on to the extent that it is and I think, like most of us, he is happy with the status quo because it suits him. But, if you talk to him he is a very, very responsive person.
Sycamore	If you just met him in the corridor, you could have picked up the case and talked about it?
Beech	Yes.
Sycamore	You couldn't at that stage but you might now.
Mahogany	The chances of meeting him in the corridor are very small but . . .
Beech	Yes. A very approachable man.
Mahogany	So it *was* your, I can't remember, 'collusion amongst the women . . . ' (referring to Dr Bourne's phrase, in a previous session)
Beech	Yes.
	(Laughter)
Bourne	What I am wondering is whether it is still continuing, I mean does he *know*? You said he didn't know and I am wondering whether he still doesn't. Does he know? Or is he still kept in the dark, by you?
Beech	I don't know. How do you mean?
Sycamore	About the superintendent! Did you tell him what had happened? (laughing)
Beech	I didn't, but he did describe her as a good fairy which I told him was very insulting and I thought that that possibly summed up the whole situation. He actually saw her as his good fairy, which really is just about the most insulting description that *anybody* could be described as. I think anyway. No, I was more interested in just seeing what kind of man he was and how responsive he was to physios and patients. And it was very good. But I feel now I could go straight to him, so from my point of view I feel that all the problems have been pushed aside. But for the rest of the staff I don't know.
Sycamore	It would be quite interesting to know, do you . . . are you going to be doing this clinic in the future or was it just the once?
Beech	No. But I get patients, on his notes he actually says 'Ms Beech, please treat'. And I think this is *great*, you know, the old ego goes like *this* (mimes swelling of the head).
	(Laughter)
Sycamore	But it would be quite interesting to see whether you have become involved in the collusion, sort of versus . . .
Beech	Oh I've organised it with him, when I can see him.
Voice	Yes, I wondered.
Bourne	I expect the secretary has too and so has the superintendent, I mean isn't this the point? (ie that each woman arranges something exclusive.)

Sycamore	Yes, that's what I am thinking about.
Lime	And what happens to the next person who goes?
Voice	Are you going to, say if somebody happens to talk to you about the kind of situation that happened to you, do you say, 'Oh, so and so, he's in the clinic at such and such, why don't you just go in and see him'? Or are you going to start sort of putting barriers up or ... ?
Beech	Oh no, I think the answer is that nobody really knows him, none of the other physios. They tended to not really know what he was like and when they asked me what I thought and I said that I thought he was a great guy and very amenable and very willing to discuss patients, they were very surprised. And I said, 'It is our reticence really. If you went to see him he would be more than willing to discuss the patient very fairly.' And I think they possibly might, I don't know.
Teak	What happened to the lady with the facial palsy?
	(Somebody has finally remembered the patient, lost in all this.)
Beech	Well we ... I had to chat to him very quickly about that and I hadn't treated her for a week. He had a chat with her and he explained to her that − I *think* he explained to her that − they were waiting to see what would happen and she must wait too. And I think she is off treatment and she is now under ENT with sort of check-ups from him every two months or something like that. And she seemed very happy by this.
Oak	Sorry I go back to this point, but how did you manage to do his clinic, was the superintendent ... ?
Beech	No, she offered. This is the marvellous thing. After the row she said to me ...
Oak	I see, I missed the week when ...
Beech	She finally said to me, 'Well the best thing for you to do if you feel like this is to do his clinic and get to know him'. And I did his clinic and you know, it was fun.
Oak	But the clinic she would have done herself?
Beech	Oh yes. Yes. And they did my patients for me. Which was very nice. And they have also now set aside a Wednesday morning, half an hour every Wednesday morning where physios can go and see him about patients. If they ever do.
Teak	Oh how wonderful.
Mahogany	That sounds a sensible arrangement in any circumstances.
Voices	Yes.
Bourne	Well thanks for the follow-up. I was a bit intrigued, slightly, by the business of him still not knowing.
	(The matter is obviously unresolved but there are other problems to be heard.)

74

Beech	Well I can't stir up more dirt can I really?
Bourne	No . . . But it is an intriguing situation nevertheless, of him not knowing.
Beech	Well it's unbelievable, the way they creep in and out and, (whispering) 'Excuse me Dr X, I don't want to trouble you but so and so, perhaps I can do it for you'. And there is all this *bowing* and *scraping* and *licking* of boots. I have never seen anything like it. (Laughter)
Sycamore	But he does appear to like it.
Beech	He *doesn't* like it, they are good *fairies*, you know? And he's, he's . . . Would you like to be called a good fairy?
Sycamore	It depends how it was said.
Voices	Yes, I . . . (inaudible)
Beech	But it's a bit *insulting.*
Voices	Perhaps the superintendent wouldn't mind, I mean . . . (inaudible)
Beech	I think it's insulting. It's all right at Christmastime but . . . (inaudible)
Bourne	Okay, well thanks . . . shall we go on? (to Poplar)
Poplar	Well it isn't really physio but it was just the nastiest thing I have had to do in my entire life. I was coming to work this morning, saw a person lying on the floor and I said 'I am a physiotherapist, can I help?' A woman said 'Well, I have done some nursing'. And I said, had she had a fit? No. I sort of grabbed hold of her pulses and there was a faint pulse which just suddenly stopped on me. So I just started to resuscitate, if you call it resuscitating, mouth to mouth and sternal massage. And I was there for 20 minutes on Euston tube station. No bloody ambulance came. Nobody came and just . . . All the time this feeling of helplessness. All the time I knew exactly what I wanted to do, I could just feel the pulmonary oedema coming up in her — and no suckers of course, no nothing. The bloody ambulance didn't come and didn't come and I was, you know . . . A guard came up and said 'Is all this necessary?', so I sort of gave him a job to keep him quiet. I told him to squeeze her legs hard together and keep them up which he did. And eventually a person arrived who said he was a doctor and this other nurse-girl, the girl who had said she had done some nursing, stood to one side. And he said, 'She is breathing all right but there is no heart. Keep on with the massage'. And the massage was obviously effective because her pupils were going in and out. And then the ambulance finally arrived and honestly it was 25 minutes later. We then had to get her up the steps of the tube station and into the ambulance, stopping at every flight to give more massage. The doctor got stuck outside. The ambulance men went in first

and I was still doing the massage. The ambulance man put the airway in and knocked two of her teeth down her gullet. So I then had to pull the mouthpiece out and I start to blow down the mouthpiece. I pulled the mouthpiece out and found the teeth wedged in the other end so they came out with the mouthpiece. And then we changed roles and I did the mouth-to-mouth and the doctor did the cardiac massage and this pulmonary oedema was just coming up and coming up. And you know it was like blowing a bloody bubble pipe and there was blood and bubbles everywhere and she got to hospital and she was dead on arrival.

Voices   Oh dear.
together

Poplar   And I just, you know, I was just still shaking (pause – choking back tears). I mean it's just this whole case of knowing exactly what you want to do and it isn't there. And then there was a sucker in the ambulance which sort of caused mucking around with this bloody tube and her false teeth. And she was only . . . well I placed her at her late 30s, so she could have well been younger than that because when people go blue they look ancient. And they tried for about half an hour at the hospital and I sort of stood around and they then gave up. But I just can't get it out of my mind, just feeling this chest, you know, as you bounce up and down and just sort of feeling it and just trying to blow through all these bloody bubbles everywhere. And I came out and I was absolutely covered in blood. I washed my hair at work just from this pulmonary oedema. And just *not getting* anywhere. And there's just . . . well I don't know (sighs). (Pause) But if it happened in a hospital – it was just brought home to me, when I got into the hospital and everybody leapt to and they dialled 456 and everything was done fantastically well. And they were, as we would be under the circumstances, not laughing and joking obviously, but you know, they had time to say, 'My God, you look hot', and things like that. And it's just how involved you are terribly when these things happen in the street. I didn't know this woman from Adam and then sort of coming into the hospital and they were so sort of separate. I mean they were fantastically good but they were so separate. But I am just sort of so tied up in this and if it had happened in a hospital . . . I have given massage once before for a very short time in a hospital and it didn't mean much. I mean I was a student and I got excited by it but this is . . . I am just so *involved* in it. (Pause)

Sycamore   Do you think if they had got there quicker?

Poplar   If they had got there quicker and equipment had been in the room she would have been all right because every time I banged down, her pupils dilated and contracted and it was working.

76

And, as I said, she was breathing on her own and she *almost* regained consciousness, so much so that her eyes rounded and she looked at me. And I . . . you know how you speak to unconscious patients, I said, 'Okay love, you just fainted'. I don't know whether she understood, she probably didn't. But she was moving her fingers and we were doing fantastically for the first ten minutes. It seemed like two hours. But, I had looked at the clock when I came up and then I checked and looked at my watch when I got to the hospital and they asked me, you know, how long I had been doing it for. But at the time you obviously don't think about these things. I mean when you are doing ultra-violet to wounds you don't think 'Yug', but now I just sort of can't. You know, the idea of those frothy bloody bubbles all over the place which went all over me and I have still got blood on my trousers and sort of blowing into her mouth in that state and everything . . .   And I feel as if I want to clean my teeth 500 times and have hot showers, as well as the whole (inaudible). It's like kissing a dead person which it was in fact (sighs). And she was done for, the moment the ambulance arrived.

(The feelings and anxieties connected with disgust were not taken up. Some seminar leaders would have attended more closely to this theme of physical revulsion. It is particularly important to note the link Ms Poplar makes, in passing, with other physiotherapy (ultra-violet to wounds). The hint is that there is comparable disgust at other times but it is more easily suppressed during routine clinical work.)

Voices	Umm.
	(Long pause)
Voice	But still it isn't a physio problem, it's probably out of place.
Voice	Yes.
Voice	Yes that's true.
Lime	It *is* (a physio problem).
Poplar	And being the only person there who knew what was happening until this doctor came, it was me all the time. And this bloody stupid man with his cloth cap on with his 'Guard' written on it saying, 'Are you sure all this is necessary?' (Mimics his voice.)
Sycamore	Well I think you did incredibly well.
Voice	Yes.
Oak	Who did you send to summon an ambulance, not a guard?
Poplar	Well I said, 'Has an ambulance been called?' And then after a few minutes I said to the guard, you know, 'Look, go and phone again, and ask them to bring a resuscitating ambulance' because I know there is one which has got resuscitation equipment in it.
Voice	Umm.
Poplar	And I felt fairly competent about defibrillating or whatever it was. I mean you can't do any harm under such circumstances

but as I said, she *drowned* in the end. You know it was oedema.
It was, you know, like a bubble bath, like a bloody bubble bath.
(Pause) As I said, she was probably late 30s, might even have
been younger.

Voice   Umm.

Voice   Yes.

(Pause)

Sycamore   The worst thing about it was that it wasn't hopeless was it?

Poplar   It *wasn't* hopeless, no. Because at the beginning somehow, you
know, I could *feel* the massage was doing some good. I could
feel that this, first of all when this nurse started doing, (well
she said she had done some nursing) mouth-to-mouth, it wasn't
working. And then we got the head further back and you could
feel it was working and every time you pushed the pupils dilated
and the colour came, and it was working beautifully. But then
it's just like a train running down hill, things seemed to happen
going up those damned steps as well.

Voice   Umm.

Poplar   And it was virtually on the steps that things happened and in
the ambulance they couldn't find the sucker and then getting
the teeth out of the tube and out of the gullet and . . .

Sycamore   That's the point, if they had been five minutes early, she might
well have been all right.

Poplar   But I must say it was probably unusual from my point of view
because it is the first time I have ever seen anybody who is dead
except when they are laid out with a neat cover on them.

(This is an admission of the utmost importance. Physiotherapists are in
constant proximity to death but may be seriously impeded by never actually
seeing anyone dead. The problem is discussed on page 45.)

(Long pause – one minute)

Poplar   Anyway, they say it always helps to say things don't they?

Voices   Umm.

Poplar   So it's got it off my chest anyway.

(The seminar has a clear option to leave the subject there and hear another
case.)

Oak   Did the nurse come?

Poplar   No she didn't because this doctor was coming up the escalator
and he had arrived just a few minutes before the ambulance did.
He was the one who gave encouragement and said, 'Carry on, the
massage is working'.

Voices   (Something inaudible – people talking together)

Poplar   It's emotionally and physically . . . I was *dripping* with sweat.

Voices   Yes.

Teak	When a patient dies in hospital with all the (inaudible) . . .
Voices	Yes. Umm.
Beech	And also the contact.
Poplar	And then there were no doctors. Well I mean they came damn quickly but I mean they were about three minutes in Casualty with, you know, nobody there. And, of course, the 'arrest thing' was down the corridor as usual. (Pause) Anyway. (She is referring to cardiac arrest resuscitation equipment.) (Pause)
Bourne	I was just wondering whether you were partly calling into question the business of whether it *is* better to say things, because in a way what is also emphasised in this is some feeling of how maybe it's all very much *worse* if you are not in your white coat and all that.

(The seminar leader has decided not to accept the option that Ms Poplar offered, viz that she was adequately served by the chance to 'get it off my chest anyway'. Indeed, the notion is directly challenged. The whole purpose of the seminar can really be questioned: perhaps it would be better if people remained firmly in traditional roles and even talked less.)

Voice	Umm.
Bourne	And I suppose a lot of our activity here is really to get out of the white coat and in a way it is the sort of risk we run a bit in a seminar of this sort. Is Ms Poplar saying, you know, we are all going to end up in tears if we go on really . . . sort of . . . eroding our usual defences and the usual arrangements and things. It seems to me to be that sort of anxiety that's being raised too, that if we really feel, . . . start seeing through ourselves as you . . .
Poplar	Well if it comes to a happy end, does it matter? But I mean if this patient was even on ICU (Intensive Care Unit) obviously it would be OK. But it is just the fact that she is dead, that makes it so . . . I mean whatever trauma you go through it doesn't matter.
Bourne	Well that's anothing thing. I thought you were also saying that for the time being, it can look lovely. Your case, you know, sounds lovely (to Ms Beech), but I think Ms Poplar is also then reminding us of that other feeling. You know, 'It may sound lovely but really look what you are up against!' Death and . . .

(The point being raised is that the two cases, appearing so different on the surface may, at depth, involve similar horrors. Most medical people would rarely think of a facial palsy as a threat to life. The discussion now continues for several pages, juxtaposing the two cases and contrasting humdrum physiotherapy with the life-saving satisfactions of surgery.)

Beech	But that case wasn't lovely.
Bourne	No, well, Ms Teak also reminded us about that too. Actually the woman is quietly left with . . .

Poplar	That's right.
Teak	I would like to go on about that a bit, you know, from what I wanted to say last week.
Poplar	Umm, could I, if we are going back, could I have a recap of what happened in this case? (Inaudible – people laughing) (Ms Poplar was away when it was discussed before.)
Bourne	No!!

(It felt like being asked for a recap on *The Brothers Karamazov*.)

(More laughter – inaudible comments)

Poplar	Did she have a facial palsy which was left?
Beech	No it was treated daily with IDC.
Oak	And I too missed one session so . . . (people laughing – inaudible)
Poplar	And she didn't respond?
Lime	No, but she had been told that she was going to get better.
Poplar	And she wasn't, was that it?
Beech	Sorry?
Poplar	What was it that she had? A facial palsy from which she wasn't going to get better? It was a Bells?
Beech	She had, she's had, nobody really knows. Nobody can find any reason for her palsy.
Poplar	But it won't get better now, you are beyond the critical stage?
Beech	The point of the discussion was that it was, in the beginning, intimated that she was going to get better very quickly.
Voice	Umm.
Beech	And slowly the factor was introduced that she might not get better as quickly as she thought. She expected improvement day by day.
Voice	Umm.
	(Pause)
Beech	I really can't go through all that again!
	(Pause)
Sycamore	And Ms Beech had a row with her superintendent about trying to see the doctor was it?
Voice	Why did you want to see him, to explain to her that it was a slow . . .
Beech	Well because he was seeing her and he kept re-ordering this bloody IDC every day, and it was giving her a false impression of the situation. And I wanted to see him to see what his views were about IDC as to whether he felt that it could be cut down or perhaps why it was being done at all. (Pause) And the result was that the, the resulting traumas that happened caused waves which rather shook me. The actual achieving . . . the final sort of seeing the doctor caused incredible trauma . . . all round.

80

Poplar   What, to you or to other people?

Beech   Well it caused trauma to other people and I was rather staggered
           at the actual trauma it caused. And so, although on one side of
           it one felt a feeling of satisfaction that you had got the result,
           you know, that you had actually got to see the doctor and . . .
           the other side of it was that (pause) . . . that the trauma, and the
           um, I can't explain it . . . I was shattered actually that it had so
           many repercussions as it had.
           (Pause)

Bourne   What were your, what were your angles on it? (to Ms Teak)

Teak   After the last time we spoke about it I had tea in the orthopaedic
           clinic on the Friday, I raised this whole business. I said I spend
           my life going on a Wednesday afternoon to a seminar, at which
           there was a great interest you see, at the Tavistock. And then I
           said it is difficult to convey the whole atmosphere of the seminar
           and what we are here for. But I did come concrete and cited
           this case that Ms Beech was treating, this particular patient with
           the facial palsy and the daily treatment by IDC and the impossi-
           bility or seeming impossibility of speaking to the man who
           ordered it. That seemed to me the crux of the situation. Well
           we went on about this. Now Dr X says, 'I think it is iniquitous
           that a physiotherapist hasn't got access to the person who orders
           the treatment, free access to speak to anybody responsible'. And
           we raised the question of saying to the patient, whose responsible,
           whose job it is to say, 'Look! This is a pretty useless' — well not
           quite so bluntly, but, 'It isn't a treatment that's going to cure
           your Bell's palsy', if you like. The feeling amongst the clinic
           was that it is not the job of the physiotherapist to convey that.
           Nor is it the job of the physio to undermine a treatment that is
           ordered, but it is the job of the physio to go to the person res-
           ponsible and say what she or he thinks about the treatment
           ordered and where they are getting, and this needs free access.
           The registrars say that we in our hospital have this good liaison.
           If a physio comes and says, 'Look I think that's pretty useless
           and for this, that and the other reason . . . ' Fine. And they do
           agree that in other hospitals it isn't so. People are asked to do
           treatment and there isn't this exchange of opinion. But they
           think that it is up to the physio not to do a bilgey treatment
           and to say, you know, stick to your guns. And this business of
           the superintendent physio making it difficult for junior staff to
           get near the big chief is an iniquitous situation which certain
           people do perpetuate. And then I mentioned this thing which
           you (Dr Bourne) said about collusion of women — I don't know
           whether I quoted that right — about the collusion of women.
           Do the women, do we perpetuate this situation? Where we
           make the big chief so sort of inaccessible to ourselves and the
           patient? But we go on doing things that we don't *believe* in.

	And then it opened up the whole question, I said something about job dissatisfaction, and bilgey treatment. So, it is generally agreed, I mean saving your presence (to Ms Poplar) that we are not in a life-saving job.

Poplar   It didn't work.

Teak   No, but *we* are not really in a 'life-saving' job, and that is why this is their feeling. And these are, quotes, question marks, quotes I mean. And this is their feeling — we are not, (and don't we know it!) but we are not 'essential' to the set-up.

(One or two surprised exclamations)

Teak   Then we went on to the essential ingredients in the situation, it's the doctor, the patient and the nurse really isn't it? But it *is* I think the thing of allowing ourselves to always be in this position of subservience. They think we are in a subservient job and that nurses who can't stand being in a subservient job take up medicine.

Poplar   But do you mean subservient in the fact that we are not involved with the quantity of life but we are involved with the quality?

Teak   No, no, we are subservient in the sense that we take our instructions from someone else.

Poplar   But do we?

Beech   Well, do we?

Sycamore But they have just told us not to do things we don't believe are right. I mean they want their cake and eat it, they really . . . Or they appear to be putting it that way.

Teak   It isn't quite like that. Is it cut and dried? Not . . . Nobody would suggest and I hope that I am not suggesting that when somebody asks you to treat this chap, you say, 'Well I am not going to do it because I think it is bloody useless'. That is not my intention to say that. No. That's not what I'm trying to convey. What I am trying to convey if you want the concrete example is that if you are asked to do an IDK daily, whether you do it or not, you could say at the outset or fairly soon on, what you thought about it and what you know about it from your own experience.

Poplar   Yes but there is also the problem by the hierarchy that if you opt out of doing something for *very* valid reasons, it usually gets put down to, she wants a long lunchtime or, poor girl, she has got too much work to do. It depends how Christian they are. Because I have refused to walk some D & Cs post-op. (D and C: dilatation and curettage of the womb, a commonplace minor gynaecological procedure.)

Voices   Oh my God (general laughter).

Poplar   And somebody said . . . and I you know, just chortled and I said, 'Well I have got much more work in the top ward'. In

	actual fact I didn't. But I didn't want to get into a situation where every single D & C has to be marched up and down.
Teak	But maybe you should say at the outset, 'Look this isn't a treatment'. Maybe you shouldn't be sort of landed in a situation as of saying, 'Well I am too busy'. Maybe you should come clean and say, *'Look, this is not a treatment'.*
	(Several voices in agreement)
Poplar	Yes. I entirely agree. But in the case of somebody who is terribly shaky on their feet let's say after a D & C for some unknown reason. If the nurses think that she wants to be walked and they ask a physio to do it and the physio says No, if they are that convinced they will then walk the patient themselves. And in many cases the nurses are busier than we are. I mean it doesn't always happen. Sometimes they are,sometimes they aren't.
Voices	Umm. Yes.
Poplar	But once they have got this peculiar idea into their heads, it is very difficult to get it out of them.
Voices	Umm.
	(Pause)
Teak	Well I think . . . life being what it is and the human situation being what it is I know there will always be these conflicts between us, but I think under general principles it could be laid down that I am not walking the post-D & Cs because I don't think it is a necessary form of treatment.
Poplar	Yes. Of course that is a thing which somebody else will do but of course if it is for an IDC then it is a different thing.
Mahogany	Well what was his opinion of it? I mean presumably he knew it wouldn't do any good. Why did he order it?
Sycamore	It's a sort of automatic thing to do.
Poplar	I must say I am confessing my ignorance here but I would have thought if she has got no muscular contraction and she is going to get it back eventually, what are you going to do? . . . I know it isn't going to increase the muscle strength or anything but you have got to keep, you know, the tone of the muscle, the nerves patent and all that cobblers. I mean how do you do it?
Mahogany	Don't bother! You get the same recovery whatever you do.
Poplar	Do you, genuinely?
Voice	Yes.
Poplar	Even after six months?
	(Voices in agreement)
Voice	They either (inaudible) recover or they don't.
Voices	Yes. Yes.
Poplar	You don't get anything like adhesions or anything peculiar?

83

Voice	No.
Voice	(Some inaudible)
Oak	I don't think . . .
Poplar	Has this been proven?
Voice	Yes.
Voice	Has it?
Teak	And how!
	(Various voices together – inaudible)
Poplar	I would not do it once a week but I would certainly . . .
Mahogany	(Inaudible) . . . and teach the patient massage.
Teak	It has proved to be useless. It really has.
Voice	Has it?
Mahogany	Terribly time-consuming as well (laughing).
Bourne	We are getting another dimension aren't we? Behind the question of collusion of women and all that business, which is one element in it all, what's being emphasised today is this business of death and the hopes and disappointments about treatments. It seems to me what we are really hearing here is something about why people go on doing useless treatment because it's something to do with facing our helplessness, facing the fact that people die and facing the fact that physiotherapy, like psychotherapy, is for the most part not a life-saving thing. There may be rare moments but clearly it isn't most of the time like that. But the point that has been brought out it seems to me, that nevertheless that sort of hope does lie behind it; that when you are giving somebody something for Bell's palsy *is* it all mixed up in your mind with giving cardiac massage and resuscitating the dead?
Poplar	I can see his point actually, with a view to this lady this morning, because I had done everything I could and I got involved in that patient and I went back in to see her again after my cup of tea, you know and they said, 'Well you know, it's no good. We are not getting a thing', and I said, 'Look, don't give up too early'. I said, 'I didn't. I sweated my guts out, you do something.' And sort of making a joke out of it and they laughed and said, 'Okay, for you dearie we'll try once again'. I can see that perhaps this chap . . . this chap . . . (ie the consultant in Ms Beech's case) rather liked this woman, and thought, 'Well she's an attractive woman, it's going to be sad if she gets a saggy face. Perhaps something *can* be gained by the IDC'. If you have got the *minutest* little bit of doubt in your mind and somebody else isn't going along with you, you know, it's like being enthusiastic about something and somebody says, 'Well I don't know if it's going to work'.

84

Teak	There was another point. I forgot to add that Dr X said that if whoever it was, orders the treatment and says to the physio-therapist, 'Look, she is in a sort of worked-up state and I think it will probably do her good to have this treatment, not that I expect much to happen from it . . . '
Mahogany	Yes, yes.
Teak	Not only this particular woman but we do get these situations.
Voice	You feel you want to do something for her even if its . . .
Teak	Yes, yes, yes.
Poplar	And you come up. I mean this chap might have thought that the physio was a block. Just as we think that the secretary and (inaudible) was a block.
Teak	But you see, there should be this liaise where he said that.
Voice	But in this situation it isn't like me at the X Hospital where the chap will bump into me with the slip and tell me. This is writing a slip out to an anonymous physiotherapist in the physio department.
Teak	Well, this is what's so awful isn't it?
	(Voices together − inaudible)
Bourne	This again leads back to the same thing: some things are better left *unsaid*. Perhaps it gives us a glimpse of why so much is done with little slips of paper, because if you meet face to face . . .
Voice	You have to put it into words.
Bourne	Yes, you might have to . . . it might come out that neither of you really think it's worth doing whereas if bits of paper go backwards and forwards, it may be possible to maintain the illusion.
Voice	Especially if you are trying to kid a patient because then it is not a double bind, is it? I mean if you know that it's useless and you know that *he* thinks it is useless . . .
Beech	But this is one of the great problems, you know. When I was doing my clinic and I saw new patients and old patients coming in, particularly new patients, and I saw the conversation in the office, the whole sort of development of the consultation and the situation that they arrived at, you know, to the decision of treatment and what he told the patient, and then you see that card that's written up, and you pick that card up. Somebody else picks it up and they see six words.
Mahogany	Yes.
Teak	I agree with that, yes.
Beech	You see there is no link-up.
Sycamore	But I am afraid this happens even when the physios are writing cards up. Because the physios write the cards up for most of the clinics I get cards from and this same thing tends to happen. There are a few where it doesn't and there is a bit of extra guff

85

	on the card which helps a bit. But sometimes, you know, people who know this person has a long history of, say, RA (rheumatoid arthritis) and diagnoses 'RA – Treat wax for hands'.
Voice	That's right, yes.
Sycamore	Whereas I know very well whoever was in the clinic knows that this person has a fairly long history and that some of this may surely be relevant to the present treatment. It isn't just when a clerk or somebody is writing the card. It does happen when the physiotherapist is writing the card too.
Beech	You see I had a patient this morning and they actually phoned me up about him. That phone call took two seconds and yet what they told me in two seconds was about the man, not particularly his physical state but his mental state and his whole attitude. Now I feel, I felt that when I met this man I was on a stronger basis for applying my treatment in a different way, not particularly what I did but the method in which I approached him, and that took two single seconds of a phone call. And yet, if I had just seen, 'short wave and traction' to this guy I would have just done that and thought he was like, you know, off the conveyor belt. And it would have taken me a lot longer to have discovered what was going on.
Voice	Umm.
Beech	That was just a very quick phone call with about half a dozen sentences.
Poplar	Yes this is what I mean when I say it is easier to say things than it is to write them.
Lime	So which ones does one communicate about?
Voice	The ones with the problems!
Oak	I make a point when I know there is a new physiotherapist and I see the consultant at regular intervals, I make a point sometime before to find out whether she has met him. And I often hear them say, 'Oh, he's not approachable'. And I say, 'Well come and meet him and see what happens', and I introduce the physiotherapist to the consultant.
Mahogany	Umm . . . that's nice actually.
Oak	And quite often it's to our mutual surprise that he is so approachable and she could make contact with him.
Voices	Umm. Yes.
	(Pause)
Bourne	It generally sounds better on balance to do that sort of thing but . . . I find myself wondering, about this other side of it, whether there is . . . you know, what are the advantages that keep some of these other systems going? Because there must be a considerable pay-off in doing things in a way which seems to be much more uncomfortable.

Oak	Well later on they probably communicate with just writing the requests to each other.
Bourne	Umm. I mean a lot of things which go on supposedly to save time . . . don't.
Sycamore	Or they save the very minimum of time.
Bourne	Or they save terribly little and that isn't really the explanation. But there must be some sort of pay-off about maintaining any illusions . . . The other thing that struck me I was also wondering really about, about the certain pay-off in keeping somebody to blame.
Voice	Yes.
Bourne	I mean I am thinking about your story (to Ms Poplar). It's bitterly frustrating but there is quite an appeal about the sense that if it hadn't been for the bloody ambulance man or somebody's incompetence or something like that . . .
Poplar	Oh no, I didn't mean that at all. I just meant they were probably quite legitimately out on another call. But it's just, at the time I just kept thinking . . .
Bourne	But there is something about that. 'What I could only have done if the facilities had been right!' There is quite a premium then in not having the facilities right. Because one can always bask in the dream of what one would have done if the facilities had been right.
Poplar	Yes . . . Yes perhaps it is only a dream but I would have given my eye teeth for a sucker.
Bourne	To put it another way, 'If only we were doctors or surgeons or something, unless you are unlucky enough to be a psychiatrist what life you would save!' Something of that comes into it. (Somebody laughs)
Oak	So what is it? Is it not being realistic when we think that the grass is greener on the other side of the fence?
Voice	Or wanting a let-out.
Sycamore	If only we had known this patient was such and such, if only they had written it on the card, then it would not have taken us two weeks to notice that the wrist is absolutely stiff or something. (Laughter)
Poplar	Because if only I could have read the word Arthrodesis I would not have tried to mobilise it!
Voice	Yes, exactly. (Laughter)
Voice	Well, it is human nature, this is just (inaudible).
Bourne	Maybe it is but I am just really struck by the way it is sort of brought into the working arrangements and attitudes and the sort of . . .

87

Teak I would like to go on to what I was saying about this before and that is, when we had finished this talk about our situation and so on, I did say, 'Well what is it like to be a consultant? What is it like to be a registrar? Do you feel dogsbodies like we do? Do you get your . . . what sort of satisfactions and dissatisfactions?' I mean the human lot I suppose, being the same wherever you happen to be placed in it, in a way. I (pause) . . . In the end you do feel that when you see them being involved in things that you know you couldn't do in a million years, you do get your dissatisfactions. I think this is where mine stem from, I can't speak for anyone else. I am sure of that. I am not sure of anything really but, it wouldn't be true to say that. But I feel that a lot of one's own dissatisfaction does stem from the fact that . . . as you say people doing surgery or this, that and the other, life-saving and so on, not necessarily life-saving but quality and quantity of work, terrific amount of work, terrific number of patients and terrific stuff really and sometimes you think you, well, play a very minor role in all this don't you?

(Dr Bourne has been calling attention to the temptations: (a) to maintain poor communication so as to mask awkward facts; (b) to maintain grievances so as to preserve thoughts of 'if only . . . '; (c) to idealise doctors, as life-savers. Ms Teak may now be reasserting a reality about medical achievement or she may be reasserting an idealisation. Throughout all this, we are struggling with the undercurrent of doubt about the possibility of doing anything worthwhile by mere talking. The next remarks are related to this.)

Beech I don't know except that one thing I have found since being a on the course, I have changed my attitudes and I find that instead of doing conveyor belt physio I begin to sort of try and look at the individual patient as an individual and so, I suppose in terms of pay-off in sort of satisfaction, occasionally, you get a satisfaction of feeling that the contact with the person is greater now than if I had treated him a year ago. Because I have actually made a slight effort to understand him in his situation as a human being and not just as a sort of, a patient who has got whatever is written on the dotted line by diagnosis. So that is a satisfaction in a way.

Teak Yes, I'm sure that's true.

Poplar I think also perhaps your point again is that you take somebody on the table who has got acute appendicitis and the appendix is in the pot and a couple of days later they are doing very nicely thank you. But with us, because it takes so much longer in most cases (except the good old Maitlands, which I think is a miracle working, (laughing), that's why I love it so!) It is all so much slower isn't it? I mean, miracles didn't take six months did they? I mean it happens like *that* (clicks fingers).

Voice Exactly.

Poplar I meant the original ones.

Beech	I think we're being too cut and dry. If you sit in the ortho-paedic clinic or any other clinic there is *very* little . . . I am sure a doctor must gain very little satisfaction. Surgery is only a reparative, it's a repairing thing. It isn't putting something new in its place. It's not. It's just vaguely helping somebody who has got a stiff toe by giving them, whatever. But it isn't actually giving them a brand new toe.
Teak	They do get a lot of spare parts.
Beech	No, but my point is that it isn't perfection, and we are trying to see it in too black and white terms. I don't think they get any . . .
Teak	Well that's it, I don't think there are as you say, black and white terms.
Beech	So if you think about it, do they really get any more satisfac-tion than we do, or is it just because we basically feel the under-dog and so are looking for excuses?
Teak	Well I think we *are* in an under-dog situation, I don't think anything changes that very much. I think we are in a subservi-ent role. Yes, I do.
Beech	But we are in a subservient role because we put ourselves there, (pause) because, individually, if you go to doctors they will treat you as a respectable physiotherapist. And it works from there.
Poplar	I hate to raise the old subject up again but I think it is mainly to do with the fact that still most doctors are males and most physios are females.
	(Laughter)
Poplar	And I am sure that this is the crux of the matter. I am sure it is. I mean quite honestly a good physio . . .
Bourne	It might be the crux of the matter but I do think you are side-stepping something, you know, which is, which is wearing us down a bit, this feeling about the hopelessness of the work and its uselessness.
Beech	No, she didn't say that surely.
Bourne	I think this is the point. I think in a way people have been saying it and I haven't heard because if you go back a bit there was a notion, the basic collusion wasn't it, was between all the women, physiotherapists, *not* to inform the doctor. And, as you emphasise it isn't just a matter of grumbling and binding, but really *informing* him and showing him that, look, this treatment is *really* useless and no progress is being made. Now in a way I find myself wondering, is this really what you are saying; that there is this collusion going on here, that in a similar way I am being protected from really being met with the full force of your anger and hopelessness about the work you do, as well as maybe the work of the seminar. Did that woman

89

on Euston station live half a minute longer by virtue of the work in this seminar? And anyway, as you say apologetically, it wasn't physiotherapy, you know. The moment of glory was not physiotherapy. I know it's come up from time to time that the work is not proven and it is all empirical and so on but I wonder if we really have plumbed the depths of despair and whether I have been rather protected from it.

(This type of transference interpretation is uncommon in these seminars. In every discussion of a transcript we reach the point where some people feel that the seminar will not be able to get on with its work until the here-and-now transference problem has been exposed. Others would still feel that the physiotherapists' feelings of gloom and futility in their own work is *not* better understood by linking it up with similar feelings about the work of the seminar. The fact that we lost Ms Beech, following this session, might be taken to indicate that even more attention should have been paid to the anxiety and gloom within the seminar itself — but the argument always goes both ways. There is really no reason to decide, necessarily, that it would have been better (or *for whom* it would have been better) if she had stayed. It hurts the seminar leader to lose members but perhaps he should just put up with it.)

Poplar	What, despair in the sessions or despair in our jobs?
Bourne	Both.
Voice	Both.
Lime	Umm . . . I know it's something I only resolved because I felt it very early and perhaps it was while I was still a student, very deeply, dissatisfaction with what I was expected to do and how I was not expected to talk about the things that I thought mattered. And I suppose I worked it out through joining an organisation which is off-beat as far as thoughts were going on then, as far as health service work was concerned. And very much thinking of it or of reconciling it sort of more as an educational process. But this might be just my own way of balancing out, and very much thinking of it . . . actually sort of coming to the Tavistock to the seminar last year, you know, trying to find for myself the larger concepts of what I was doing, or what I could hope to do. But it helped, you know . . .
Poplar	I must say I felt this very much about being the small very minor cog in a very very big wheel which was why I have opted to be the queen bee in a very small hive. But I thought it was the physio set-up where you had, you know, the hierarchy going down, because I opted out very early on. I would blame it on the physio system, I still do. I don't blame it on the fact that some people are doctors and some people are physios, at all.
Teak	What do you blame on the physios then?
Poplar	The feeling that you are . . . not as important as some people, that if you want to talk to somebody up in the hierarchy you have got to ask a senior who then asks the superintendent who

90

	then talks to the doctor, and so on. And as I said I didn't blame it on being *a* physio, I just blamed it on the, you know, the grande dame physio system.
Teak	Isn't that what you (Dr Bourne) are calling the collusion of women?
Bourne	Well except that I see it now as a link to something else, which is the maintaining of an idea of somebody who is sufficiently high up, like God Almighty, to resuscitate the dead. (Pause) There seems to be that sort of, um . . . On the one hand there is a very immediate sort of despair and sense of futility about a lot of things but what resuscitation is going on up there! I mean the surgeons who save a life a minute.
Poplar	Yes I entirely and completely and utterly agree.
Sycamore	And the reverse of the coin — they do destroy a life a minute, I mean they're not . . .
Bourne	In reality there may be all sorts of things but I mean in some way I get the sense that people may be inflamed much more. I don't think it's the overt idea. We can all be blasé about surgeons and, you know what orthopaedic operations are like half the time and so on. But there is some *underlying* idea of a treatment which really works and resuscitates.
Teak	I mean one way and another we are voicing dissatisfaction aren't we? Of some sort or another. Or trying to understand ourselves.
Voice	(Inaudible)
Teak	What about when you talk about resuscitating and so on when we verify that when you and I very first came to this I seem to remember the patient of Ms Elm's (referring to Case 44), this patient with the Parkinson's that nobody dared name as Parkinson's. It seems to me *always* that we are involved in some peculiar set-up aren't we? Something a bit ; . .
Voice	That's a bit strange isn't it?
Voice	Yes.
Voice	Very peculiar.
Teak	As though we have to maintain something we don't *believe*.
Voice	Yes.
Voice	Umm.
Teak	In some peculiar way we are involved in maintaining a situation or a myth or a . . .
Lime	But isn't that because . . . because we are trying to maintain it in some way.
Teak	Well are we?
Lime	Well I wonder.
Teak	I don't know. Is this the human lot — I mean does everyone

	indulge in this sort of . . . does everybody find themselves in this situation whatever his calling, so to speak?
Bourne	I suppose the problem is a bit to try to identify when we go overboard with it. I mean, as you say, obviously it is pretty prevalent, universal and all that, but . . . I think we are really getting right up to the end of the garden path with it.
Sycamore	Perhaps when we are sitting here talking about things like our problems, they seem very enormous and big and enveloping but for Heaven's sake we are still all *doing* the job so we can't all be experiencing *such* enormous job dissatisfaction.

(True or untrue? Probably some were experiencing very great job dissatisfaction. Ms Sycamore herself became pregnant soon after this and will be out of physiotherapy for some time. So her job-satisfactions are certainly in for a change.)

Mahogany	I think there is a hell of a lot of it actually, more than one would . . .
Beech	I think that also physios, because of the job dissatisfaction are very sort of lethargic and lazy and they just accept their lot.
Mahogany	Yes.
Sycamore	*Or*, are we trying to make martyrs of ourselves?
Beech	Yes. I think it is self-perpetuating.
Sycamore	Yes. That's what a lot of the women I know in my life tend to do.
	(Laughter)
Sycamore	It's something I know I do myself too. But if we remain relatively calm and look at the situation about which you got frightfully steamed up, and look at it fairly quietly . . .
Mahogany	That's the trouble, we are all too quiet!
Sycamore	Too quiet?
Mahogany	Yes.
Poplar	I can truthfully say that I have no job dissatisfaction. I mean I have got specific dissatisfactions like the fact that there is nothing to do but pre and post-ops (ie exercises) and all that cobblers but I can't blame that on the place I am at and you know . . .
Mahogany	Do you get actual satisfaction in doing your pre- and post-ops?
Poplar	No, nothing so specific as that, I mean the dissatisfaction I am suffering, which I do suffer . . .
Lime	It depends what else you put into it.
Sycamore	Whether you are simply trying to physically help the patient or help the patient mentally as well.
Lime	I think this is . . . provides an excuse to go and see the patients.
Teak	Help the patient, full stop.

Beech	I think this is something that perhaps we see ourselves or have seen ourselves in the past as *physical therapists*. And I think that perhaps, I don't know, I'm not suggesting we are psychiatrists in our new role, but you know, it is quite interesting to actually look at the patient as a human being.
	(Laughter)
Poplar	But did you not do this before?
Beech	Not very much no. Not in sort of . . . No! Not as much as I in fact try to do now.
Poplar	Do you think it is more difficult in this set-up where you get four patients every half hour in the clinic? I am sure it is.
	(Pause)
Bourne	You know that it *is* possible to have a perfectly self-respecting psychological treatment which isn't rooted in the taking of a family history to three generations and all the rest of it.
Sycamore	You mean that we have trouble in recognising we may be helping someone psychologically?
Lime	We've never had any instruction in *anything* to do with this.
Voice	None at all.
Sycamore (continuing)	When we are actually sort of *pretending* to do physiotherapy.
Bourne	Well, that comes into it. Sometimes you pretend and sometimes you don't. There is some notion of really doing things which are basically psychological treatments to encourage people and get them through. I mean, half rehabilitation work is overcoming people's fears and all that.
Voice	Yes.
Bourne	It hasn't necessarily got to be based on analysing them or . . .
Voice	No.
Bourne	Or anything like that it's . . .
Voice	No, quite.
Bourne	But there seems to be . . . a sort of muddle about that.
Lime	But it's actually difficult I think. I mean, I have been involved in doing group work, you know, with ante-natal mums and I knew things went on in the group. I knew there must be more in this than met my eye. I knew it sometimes seemed to work because I saw them in the town afterwards and that the whole sort of aura seemed to be something that they appreciated. And I have had to do a *hell* of a lot of reading to find out what it is that I am doing. And to know whether it has a place. Maybe it is because I want to fit it in somewhere or to know what it is I *don't* know.
Bourne	But what I want to differentiate is the disadvantages of knowing. Sometimes I think there are, say, advantages in knowing more about groups if you are working with groups, let's say, . . . What

93

	I want to differentiate is the area in which, yes there are advantages of knowing, as distinct from some notion of, 'Oh yes, to do groups you have got to do it properly and you have got to know how it is done. You know you have got to do it like a psychiatrist would do it.'
Voices	No! No!
Bourne	No, you say that! (ie you say that now) But there *is* some idea. And really extrapolating further, there is the sense of, it is one more version of doing it like God. That is what I am slightly bothered about. I can quite . . . I want to differentiate the sense in which you actually want to pursue and need to pursue your psychological skills and learn whatever you can, if you can, here, or in any other way. But you are all mixed up with something which is quite different, which is being-bemused-with-one-more-version-of-God-Almighty. A sort of magician-expert who 'does it properly'.
Teak	Well . . .
Bourne	But like you (Ms Beech) say self-disparagingly, 'I know we are not going to be psychiatrists *but* . . . '
Beech	I thought you were going to take me up on that! (laughing).
	(Laughter)
Beech	No what I was trying to say was the job satisfaction then can be in a very much smaller sphere of a patient who has, instead of booking into a sterile department with you in your white coat and say, 'Mr Smith if you would like to go into that cubicle I won't be a moment'. And switch the thing on and say, 'Is it warm enough?' But, not to sort of have him pour out his woes and his troubles and be sort of a lay psychiatrist, but somehow to just create an ambience where he feels that it isn't *quite* the scene, the sterile scene, that he imagined, that there is a feeling of relaxation, that somebody is quite interested in him as a person.
Voice	Umm.
Beech	And that, if one could do that, there is quite a feeling of satisfaction because it is changing the image slightly. It is changing the image of the physio department, bang bang bang, there are your crutches off, you are not doing that quite right, move your left foot a bit more! It's not quite so regimental and authoritarian. But you need more time.
Voice	Yes.
Poplar	And I think in many ways it is the set-up which is preventing us from all this, both the hierarchy set-up and the clinic set-up of so many people around at such and such a time.
Mahogany	Well you can only do this if you, yes . . .
Beech	If you have got time, that's right.

Poplar	If you are on your own. Some people prefer ward work more because then you can alter it, when the patient's all ready to talk you can stay there. You are more in contact with the patients on the ward.
Lime	I can see that now. I have been back on the wards now for three weeks, it is certainly easy.
Poplar	Not only time-wise but you can get close to the patient somehow.
Beech	But don't you think that if we . . . getting away from the image - of-God sort of doctor, if we went towards the patient more, then we would have more feeling of job satisfaction in our own way. I think we are in no-man's-land at the moment.
Lime	I think also that one of our jobs is to help the patient under-stand the doctor. It sounds sort of patronising but I think if you find a patient that is sort of idealising the doctor in one way or another, they are heading for an awful cropper sometime if you can't try and make him into a human figure.
Beech	Yes but you have got to see him as a human figure before you can teach the patient too! (laughing)
Teak	When you are talking about God you don't mean our conception of the doctor, do you? I understand you to mean that we feel and I am sure I recognise myself in this picture, that 'if only I could do this bigger and better, you know, more like God does it . . .'
Bourne	Well I mean somebody who is going to resuscitate you. I mean if I go into hospital with *my* perforation I want God Almighty, I don't want some surgeon who has got problems at that point.
Voice	But you said (inaudible).
Bourne	There is something about this isn't there? That when you want your life saved . . .
Poplar	Yes, to whom do you say your prayers, God or the doctor? (Pause)
Bourne	Well, as you rightly say, it *is* a sort of banana skin because one can be awfully bemused by it and led on to all sorts of peculiar behaviour. I mean like your set-up where that guy is obviously maintained in some strange position as a supposed answer to people's needs. Got to keep everybody alive, you know, life eternal, as if the millenium is going to come in that department. It is *that* sort of thing that we believe in. A bit of magic here and there, you know, keeps us all going I suppose. But the problem is, I think, we do need to identify it when it takes us really up the creek. (Pause)
Beech	But I do wonder how readily I would go and repeat that per-formance again. Because if the situation occurred, knowing that it caused the trauma it did, I mean, the reason why I did it

	was because I wanted one thing and one was being . . . but the next time you do it you know what you are going to do and so you know, to be forewarned as to . . .
Lime	But you are not giving credit to anybody else for having learnt from that, are you?
Teak	What do you mean, do you mean confronting the superintendent? Is that what you mean?
Beech	I suppose so.
Lime	I mean things aren't ever the same, exactly the same, are they again?
Voice	No.
Mahogany	Well surely the superintendent must realise! To sort of organise half an hour to see the consultant — that's fantastic.
Lime	Yes, I think it's super.
Beech	It looks very good superficially, but underneath it all there are all kinds of undercurrents which all come out if you press the button again. That's what I am talking about. It looks lovely on the surface. But you go and press that button again and see what happens!
Mahogany	Well you can't get the sack (laughing).
Bourne	Could we, in fact, hear yours, because we have only got a quarter of an hour (to Ms Oak).
Oak	Oh, I don't know that I will put everything to you that I want to put now that I . . . but . . . I will try. Last Monday I met yet again a patient whom I met last October, who was brought in last Monday for manipulation under anaesthetic of her cervical spine. So when I saw her on Monday, they get these operations on Tuesdays and I quite often don't know who's coming for admission for these things. So I was surprised to see her and I recognised her face . . . and I knew instantly that it was her neck. Well last Monday she held her head very rigidly with eyelids dropped down and really unable to move her head. So I thought Ah, this is the same woman. She had manipulation in October and it wasn't successful. So I was giving her breathing exercises, actually following my own little routine I go and meet them, see who it is because I will be assisting with this on Tuesday afternoon. And I often get the request or a notification while I am . . . either while I am there or an hour after. But I meet them and I usually give them, make myself known, give them breathing exercises. But this time, sitting down to give her breathing exercises I thought she needed to be listened to rather than instruct her in breathing exercises because her anaesthetic was of a very short duration. (Pause) Anyway I had a very tiny talk with her. I asked how long her neck was better after the last time and she said, well as soon as she left the hospital it was stiff again, the stiffness came gently but very quickly. You know,

gently but very quickly. It very soon set on, it crept up. So I thought to myself, 'Well I will just sit here and see what else you tell me.' And I remember I asked her about her family and last time she said to me in October when she was about to go and we talked about her having a collar or not, she asked me for a collar and I said, 'As a matter of fact, the doctor doesn't want you to have a collar. Don't have a collar'. But I told her what to do and what not to do with her neck and *then* it came out that she has two children. One of her boys at 16 made an attempt on his life and she is rather . . . she was anxious. So I had that in mind when I sat by her bedside last Friday, and she didn't say much more. So I left her and soon afterwards the houseman came to take the medical history and then we all met on Tuesday in the theatre. And while we were waiting for the patient to be brought in the houseman said, 'And she was here last October', and then it clicked with the consultant that he put her on the waiting list a long time ago but by the time she is seen that is, you know, quite a long time, her neck wasn't successful. It was stiff. There was a moment of silence when I came in and I said to the consultant that I spoke to her this morning and she said to me that she is worried and does he know? Does the consultant know that she has got a son who has made an attempt on his life? And he said, 'No'. And the houseman didn't know about it. So . . . then it came out from the consultant that he will just test her neck under anaesthetic and if it is free he will not do anything and we will refer, he will refer her to a psychiatrist and he said to me, 'You find out from her whether there is something else about her son making an attempt!' And I am to tell him and then he will write the request for a psychiatrist. Well that was Tuesday afternoon, yesterday was it? This morning, again I just followed a routine. I sent my porter to bring this lady down because she is in a room, a rather small room with another patient and I thought I won't be able to check her exercises well, so she was in my Department. I said, 'Well how is your neck today?' She laid down so that she could be in comfort and I tried to move it and it was *very* stiff. She asked me whether the doctor injected it because it was injected last time. And then I thought to myself, 'Well — what am I to tell her'. You know? So I said, 'No, it wasn't injected, the doctor just moved it for you and it went from side to side'. And then she said, well she didn't think he injected it because it is as stiff today as it was all the time before. I don't know what I said then, but I just looked at her and asked her whether she works, and he did ask yesterday in the theatre, where she worked. The consultant thought that she was in an office but I had the suspicion that she wasn't and today I asked her, 'Where do you work?' And she doesn't work in an office. She works in a factory where she is assembling parts for telephones. And she is

high-sitting on it and has actually to turn her head through a
very small range but hold her arms up. And that was bringing
the pain on. I said, 'Well, after work do you feel the pain or
where does the pain go?' She didn't know where it goes away
and it comes on when she isn't at work. So I said, 'Did you
ever tell doctor about when the pain goes?' And she said, 'He
never asked'. But they always ask (ie in Ms Oak's view).

Voice   Yes.

Oak   And er, then I said, 'Well while you are talking to me, turn your
head to the right', and she was unable to turn fully and I was on
her left side. And, 'Turn to the left' and it did get past the
middle just really five degrees, just there. So I said to her, 'Stay
in this position, don't force it any more', because she was growing pink in the face. 'Don't force it, just let it be there, tell me
something, tell me things, keep talking and the gravity will
move it more to the left'. And she did and I moved my chair
slightly more to the left but just, and erm, she said to me . . .
yes I asked how was her son and she said, 'Well he is now sitting
exams.' She corrected me, he is no longer 16 years old, he is
26. She said, 'I did tell you that *when he was 16* he made an
attempt on his life but it is ten years ago'. So I said, 'What does
he do now?' 'Oh he is sitting for — he went to work for a while.
At 16 he passed 9 subjects O level and now he is back in the
college', and I asked her what he is studying. Commerce subjects.
And I said, 'Do you think he will pass his examinations?' She
thought he will be very successful and pass them with flying
colours and this is what she is worried about, because he passed
the previous examinations with flying colours and made the suicide attempt. And I said, 'Well do you think it might happen
the same?', and she said 'Yes'. So I then said, 'Well, you know,
have you never told this to the doctor?' Oh she didn't think he
would be interested. Then she said to me, quickly, her son had
psychiatric treatment for eight years, from the age of 16 on-
wards, and people used to come to her place to treat him. Two
people came to her place to treat him, and she was in the room.
And she reminded me that she had remarried twelve years ago,
a very nice man and . . . who knew her husband and her two
children whilst they were still married, and he knew how dreadful her husband was. So I listened and she told me how dreadful
her husband was. And her husband used to, well he sold the
furniture, left her — her children were two years and four years
old. The older son, who is married, lives away from mother in
Manchester somewhere and it's the younger one who is 26 now,
sitting for examinations. And they had a dreadful life with
father. He was in prison many times. She had to make clothes
for her children on a hand·machine and he used to stand behind
her with his hands around her neck saying that if this other
man would come in he will strangle her. And then she said,

'Is there any sign of damage on my neck?' So I said, 'I didn't look for it. If you think that there might have been, you never mentioned it'. She hasn't. So I then didn't know and I said to her, does she want *me* to tell the doctor, that it might throw some light on the stiffness in her neck? Or does she want to talk to him herself? And I asked her whether she has seen the doctor today, knowing that she hasn't been able to because I spoke to him in the morning and he was in a **hurry** to attend somebody else's ward round. So I said to her, 'Well, he might be able to come and speak to you this afternoon or tomorrow, and maybe you will want to tell him things'. And then I hesitated, not knowing whether I should tell *him* and say to her, 'I will tell him that you want to speak to him'. But I thought it would be much better if she could . . . And after, when I was listening to what she said, I then made up my mind to say to her that it will be better if she wanted to talk to him spontaneously, and she said to me, 'Well, will they want to listen? They are so busy'. And I said, 'They will want to listen if you want to tell them. If you don't want to say anything, no one has any moment to listen'. So I said, 'We are waiting for the head to move a little further'. And I know yesterday (ie under anaesthetic) that it went right to the left. So am I presumptuous when I think I will wait and see what she will offer the doctor tomorrow — today or tomorrow? And then tell him myself what I discovered which I know is what she wanted me to tell him. Because she told me she hasn't said that much to anybody. And she went on to say that she wasn't able to tell anybody because she didn't think anyone would understand. Her friends don't know her. She felt that if she could tell her friends how much she got . . . what her life was while she was still married to her husband they wouldn't be so hard on her as they are now. So I said, 'Well some people would and some wouldn't, it is difficult to expect everybody to understand your feelings but there are people who specialise in that'. And if she only opened to someone it might be all right. And she went on to tell me how much she suffered from her first husband. He used to beat her and the children and the young boy was two then and ran under the table to hide himself. And then I said, 'Well does he ever speak about his father now?' No, she said he doesn't, but sometimes when he laughs or so and she says, "It's just like your father", he says, "Well I wouldn't know would I?" I said well it is true he has never seen him, you know. She doesn't know where her husband is now.

Poplar   Ex (ie ex-husband).

(This is the first moment at which anybody can see a way to come in on Ms Oak's presentation, which has taken nearly 15 minutes, and we are nearly at the end of the session. Does this matter? It is interesting to note that in this final case we have, without realising it, accepted the notion proposed and rejected previously with Ms Poplar's case; we have somehow had to accept that our function must sometimes be to listen and accept, rather than to discuss and question.)

Oak	Sorry, ex-husband. And her present husband knows the story and doesn't mind, doesn't blame, he's just there. But she said at the same time she is not allowing the present husband to be head of the family. Because she does her own decorations, painting the ceiling, and . . . (Surprised laughter)
Oak	And I said, 'What, with a neck like this?' And she said, 'Yes, perhaps the stiffness of the neck is through the painting of the ceiling', and I said, 'I don't know'.
Mahogany	Oh God.
Poplar	So what sort of relationship has she got with her present husband? If she doesn't allow him to do the painting, lucky man? I mean does she talk to him, is it a sort of side by side relationship or an integrated relationship?
Oak	I don't know, you see she . . .
Bourne	I think we will have to keep this in mind for next time, we haven't left enough time — I'm sorry.
Oak	Yes.
Bourne	(Something inaudible)
Voices together	(Inaudible)
Oak	I just wanted to correct, to supplement my last Wednesday's case. When I spoke about the patient who has got a painful back, she was the physiotherapist, I think Ms Beech wasn't there, but you will remember it from the case Ms Ash reported. I didn't make it quite clear that I am treating the patient now, but Ms Ash has gone. It came out somewhere in the lift that it isn't that Ms Ash is there and I am treating the patient. She has left the hospital . . . (Voices together)
Voice	Have you (Dr Bourne) decided when Easter is yet? (Loud laughter and voices)
Bourne	I thought you were going to ask for the Resurrection! (Voices and laughing)
Bourne	But didn't we decide last week? (Voices together confirming dates)
Oak	We usually get a nice reminder from your secretary.
Bourne	Yes — I hope so. We have two more weeks and then (voices confirming) we miss three. (Voices)
Bourne	(To Ms Lime) — I'm sorry you're going.

Voice	So am I, we shall miss you.
Lime	So am I — but I hope I'll keep in touch and hear how it's all going on.
Voices	Mutual thanks — offers of lifts and farewells.

End of session.

Part II

Session notes and cases

Part II

Session notes and cases

Introduction

This section consists of the notes made by the author, the leader of the
seminar, after each session. The notes are reproduced almost exactly as
they were originally written, except for disguising names, places and
personal details. I should emphasise that the notes are highly subjective
and idiosyncratic. They were written as a private diary with no idea that
they might ever be published – except, in the way every diarist has a
sneaking eye on posterity and an imaginary audience.

In seminars, as run in this Tavistock unit, the seminar leader has to
bottle up a great deal. It is perfectly possible to run very different seminars
in which the seminar leader does indeed lead with as much of his own personal knowledge, insight, guesses and free associations as possible. Sometimes
the seminar leader finds himself forming strong opinions and, on the face of
it, it might be a simple matter for him to voice them. Actually, there are a
number of difficulties about this which have been the topic of 25 years of
debate in the Tavistock GP and Allied Professional Workshop. The problem
is that even if the seminar leader is right in all his views and does indeed
know better than anyone else in the room, everybody's reliance on this
possibility creates a climate in which work is very restricted. There is the
danger of a dependency culture in which people lose faith in their own
abilities and lack the courage to make mistakes and struggle with their
results. There is an excessive premium on 'being right' which results in
people moulding themselves in the image of the leader if they can and falling
by the wayside if they cannot. By creating an atmosphere in which everything centres around himself, the leader exacerbates one of the most troublesome trends pervading the healing and helping professions. Doctors and
allied professionals need to acquire models of work in which clients are not
sucked into a dependency culture but are actively helped to discover their
own resources.

The foregoing has been written in terms of the seminar leader 'being
right' but keeping quiet about it. He is in any case likely to be right only
part of the time and this makes a dependency culture all the more disastrous.
It is also a fact of life that whatever the leader or teacher says is going to be
given a great deal of weight, however diffident he is about it. One of the
problems of being diffident is that the little one does say assumes added

105

importance because it is produced after evident thought and hesitation.

All in all, we have to steer a course between the need to be effective and responsible consultants to groups of people working together, helping them to make the best use of their time,using all our insight to intensify the struggle with difficulties where it seems fruitful to do so and yet, on the other hand, playing a role which allows people to develop and discover themselves, and provides the model for these same therapists to resist excessive dependency in their own clients.

This is a very long preamble, indeed a piece of special pleading, to explain why the seminar leader has so much to put down on paper afterwards. There is not only the question of getting down a few notes which will provide an *aide-mémoire* to facilitate review of the work; there is also the tremendous pressure to uncork his mind and record some of the thoughts and reactions which it seemed inappropriate to voice in the seminar itself.

Notes and references, where they arise, are listed after the report of each meeting.

First meeting — Wednesday, 1st March, 1972

At first Ms Hazel was the only person to make any offer and her supervisor had very 'helpfully' gone over her lists with her to pick out some 'suitable' patients. The patient was then very quickly sketched in as passing from pillar to post amongst the doctors, with the physiotherapist unable to get the psychological problem recognised. I stopped her there and we had a bit of ventilation on the enormous uncertainty as to what is 'a suitable case' for the seminar, or for a physiotherapist, together with the second problem — the professional relationship with doctors. Bitter complaints came out regarding the way their number one problem is to get status and independence away from the stranglehold of blind doctors. But I pointed out the way I was immediately being pushed into the boss-doctor role. I had made my ignorance very explicit together with my awareness that there must be a wide range of possible cases to discuss, whereas the only thing to come forward was something picked out by a supervisor and anxiously submitted to me to be deemed suitable or unsuitable. Did they not know if they had a headache without somebody else telling them? This drew the offer of another case from Ms Oak and it later turned out that many others had cases ready to bring.

Case 1 (Ms Hazel)

A 15-year-old girl strained her back lifting a cupboard and has had backache ever since, so severe as to prevent her coping with a day at school. The doctors sent the girl to the physiotherapy department for traction, which they were reluctant to give but did. (The girl had some degree of spinal mobility — not apparently uncommon in adolescence — which would indicate muscle-strengthening treatment, if anything.) They soon stopped this and went on to a range of other treatments and this has continued, on and off, for over a year. The girl does not come over clearly but her mother is very elegant and the physiotherapist felt the mother very much in the way. Some time later in the year the girl changed her name from Susan to Phillipa and a few months ago the father had a coronary thrombosis. The girl is adopted.

There is an intense awareness of a psychological problem and a vague sense that the doctors won't see and insist on psychological management.

106

On the other hand, the physiotherapist has 'been very careful to keep the conversation entirely normal' and avoided anything that might broach trouble between the girl and her mother. Nevertheless, she (the physiotherapist) has been quite attentive and energetic in trying to help the girl, ringing the school secretary, arranging for the girl to go and help with a vet over the school holidays (she loves animals) . . . I linked this with some earlier remarks about how 'we can only help our patients if they like and/or respect us'. We may have to question this contention.

I went on to try and establish some notion of *diagnosis* by the physiotherapist as being an important part of her skill — and thence the question of whether one can diagnose anything about the sort of person one is dealing with. Is there something about this elegant mother with her daughter, with whom everything has to be kept nice? And is all the emphasis on the fatuously brittle doctors something to do with a sense of the father in the background who falls to bits with a coronary? My reference to this last point produced a swift regression to generalities and banalities so I think it was probably right.

Case 2 (Ms Oak)
A woman suffering from severe weakness and pain in the foot, following a minor injury three years ago. she fell over a board left around by her husband and there is quite a bit of grievance over this, as being his fault. After three years of half-hearted physiotherapy in the out-patients clinic, with lights being shone etc, the physical medicine doctor suddenly decided to admit her for intensive treatment. Ms Oak was clearly told there was no organic lesion but would she please treat it! She then presents herself to us as 'a very bad psychiatrist' who 'did all the wrong things' but she managed somehow to cure this woman in three weeks. It emerges later that her management was probably pretty firm, if kindly, and that the general ward situation was fairly grim, with severely disabled patients all round, and much worse. Anyhow, she forced this patient to get better and there is an atmosphere of, 'I didn't know my own strength!'

Only one voice is ready to remark on the extraordinary success of her treatment while all the others try to make her feel that she has been 'treated like a dustbin' by her medical colleague. I felt that they were trying to make her feel bad about this. I suspect that part of the trouble stems from the annoying discovery that the physiotherapist can work these miracles if the doctor tells her that she can. It was difficult to get them off the preoccupation with the idiocy of the doctor who had mucked about for three years and on to the more interesting immediate question of how this success had been achieved. I was repeatedly invited, by Ms Oak, as well as by others, to pronounce dire risks of paralysis turning up elsewhere and to pontificate about the need to get to the bottom of it all — and it is indeed a glaring fact that we have no knowledge at all what is making this woman tick. Nevertheless, I tried to focus on another differential diagnosis — was she responding to some experience of being nursed in a kindly way or was it something to do with sharp firm handling? Ms Oak was quite openly afraid of finding out anything about this woman, from her sense that she would not know what to do with any information she obtained. Others implied that they would have got her talking more, so we shall have to see and hear more of the different styles of work.

Second meeting – Wednesday, 8th March, 1972

Case 3 (Ms Sycamore)

The problem of 'whether to tell' the patient with cancer. This woman had a mastectomy 20 years ago and has developed bony secondaries during the last year. She was first referred for physiotherapy following a pathological fracture of the hip and attended Ms Sycamore's out-patient department for about six weeks until mid-January. She seemed to be depressed and weak – unresponsive to physiotherapy far beyond the disabilities they could attribute to the physical condition. Ms Sycamore found her in tears one day with the student physiotherapist treating her and, in this context, the patient asked Ms Sycamore about her own impression that, 'I think the doctor believes I have cancer and doesn't want to tell me'. Not quite a straight question but the next thing to it.

Ms Sycamore sidestepped and does not know what to do in such cases. There is no policy, no information and nobody knows what the doctors have said. The patient has been referred from the radiotherapy department – a further point underlining the likelihood that she already knows and wants to talk. Behind the recurrent complaint about the failures of the doctors (failure to explain and inform) is the relief at being able to pass this particular buck. Passing the other way, do the students land up with these cases? Hotly denied. Are these awkward patients somehow discharged, got rid of?

In the middle of all this, one member of the seminar (name unknown)[1] disclosed that her twin sister has a tumor with a bad prognosis, making the point that she has felt far better able to deal with her feelings in full knowledge than in the previous state of uncertainty. While I took this up as underlying questions about what the physiotherapist herself can take and what sort of leadership she can exert – they do have special knowledge and experience and could speak from this platform effectively if they chose – I registered inwardly my sense of the problem of anger.[2] How angry are we with these patients who embarrass us and how angry are they with us? There seemed, at one point, to be a move towards defining the proper arrangements that should exist, the proper team ('You can't do this sort of thing on your own'), the work that should be done around the family and so forth . . . but I felt that this was a flight towards some idealised notion of the happy reconciliation with death that might be (someone quoted Cicely Saunders),[3] leaping across the immediate problem of a patient who may feel bitter and inconsolable. Other questions arise about diagnosing which patients really want to know, and on what basis. Might there be a differentiation between the patient who requires to be told by somebody very peripheral to the treatment and whom they won't see again (eg the hairdresser, or ward cleaner, or the most junior nurse: all are liable to receive surprising confidences); in contrast to the person who requires to be told by a therapist who will see him through?

Case 4 (Ms Elm)

'A professional patient',[4] who has had several unsuccessful operations and is about to have another one. He lives around the physiotherapy department and resists being discharged. Somehow, Ms Elm becomes the bad person who wants to get rid of him and incurs all his emnity, while everybody else is nice, accepting him and appreciated by him. She puts her foot in it by discussing his possible discharge. She wrote to the orthopaedic consultant but he got his word in first, somehow divining the situation.

The 'orthopod' is a very nice man, unable to say no to anybody except Ms Elm and she now has the patient back. She feels her profession is being mocked and ridiculed and that resources are being misused.

Firstly, and following directly upon the cancer case, we get a very clear statement of the hatred of patients who don't get better. This angle does have to be set against the dogged work physiotherapists do for years with DS[5] patients etc but the message seemed loud and clear all the same. The other thing that came out was the question of how far this patient is one aspect of the structure of the department, where he is felt to play one person off against the other. Is this a built-in hazard of a complex department and, in particular, of supervising students? There is a feeling that the patient prefers and enjoys whatever treatment he gets from the young physiotherapists and, just possibly, getting their secret collusion, while disparaging the older woman. Certainly, the first response to the case presentation was an ingenuous reaction from a young, pretty member of the seminar (name unknown) more or less saying that *we* good-naturedly put up with these people and why are *you* so disagreeable? I missed my chance to clarify this bit. It also emerged that Ms Elm had tried to deal with this man by putting him in a group of patients but the group had disappeared. A warning to me![6]

Notes

1 ie unknown at this meeting. There are special difficulties but also special potentialities in this stage of a seminar's life, while there is a degree of anonymity which is lost later, and attitudes are still undeclared.
2 ie being myself, at that point, embarrassed, perplexed – and even somehow angry.
3 Dame Cicely Saunders – a pioneer in studying and teaching the care of the dying; pain and discomfort are attentively minimised in an ambiance of honesty, facing facts and patients helped preserve their consciousness.
4 Implying that being a patient has become a way of life. But the *double entendre* could be important, with underlying feelings about patients rooted in the professional classes – and patients who are disturbing reflections of ourselves.
5 Disseminated sclerosis.
6 A warning that the seminar may not find it possible to function as a group containing awkward people.

Third meeting – Wednesday, 15th March, 1972

Case 5 (Ms Beech)

A Syrian young man has come to London to combine a holiday (??) with physiotherapy for pains in the head and neck. He is getting this treatment privately and Ms Beech works privately with a doctor who appears to be some sort of specialist in the field. She explained to him that she was going to pull his neck and this produced a scene of intense panic but, after reassurance, they were able to get on with it. He made some progress and she felt that, by studying trick movements, she was able to diagnose that the physical disability had been cured and that there was now only a residual psychological component. She pressed on with the treatment but then decided she could get no further. She told him to go off and return to see her before going home. He did so a few days later and appeared remarkably improved.

The discussion seemed to get stuck on the question of how to 'manage' the administration of a treatment that frightens the patient. Nothing was discussed about its indications or efficacy, with no word of diagnosis beforehand — until I pointed this out. Thereupon, there was the pretence that everybody had taken the diagnosis for granted — a slipped disc in the neck — but on further discussion this was far from clear. Ms Beech was, for practical purposes, reasonably clear about the diagnosis on which the work was based but the real doubts were projected and buried in the seminar discussion, I thought. These doubts concern charlatanry and frightening treatment. This latter point interested me most and the physiotherapists' own remarks disclosed fantasies about public executions in Syria. Why does he have to come all the way to London to have neck traction?

Another point — this business of patients who show progress by the ability to move and then go back on it and become all stiff. This, I felt, was exactly what the physiotherapists were doing in the seminar — showing the ability to move more freely in their thoughts and fantasies but then withdrawing and covering it over with an exaggerated stiffness in the mind.

I tried to put this to them but made a bit of a mess of it. I did, more successfully I think, get across the idea that some treatments may work *because*, rather than in spite of, the fact that they are frightening and fulfil the ideas of threat and punishment. It was also possible to link this with the experience of being charged and mischarged fees — a more muted form of threat or punishment.

Case 6 (Ms Ash)
This is a patient who is herself a physiotherapist, although she has not practised for 10 or more years. The symptoms seem to be something like sciatica, with back pains going into the leg. However, it is all rather mysterious. Nobody can make a firm physical diagnosis and the impression is that Ms Ash has to treat this woman for functional or hysterical disabilities — somehow to get her moving. Actually, Ms Ash feels very uneasy about this and thinks there probably is some physical lesion there. At least once, she noticed a marked temperature difference between the two legs. I note silently the failure to proceed with this observation on a professional basis, following it up, testing it out for any recurrence — or even discussing it with anyone. Our discussion was, unfortunately, only about 20 minutes on this one and the chief emphasis was on our impression that Ms Ash had particular difficulties over this woman being a physiotherapist herself. The patient tended to 'co-operate' in an exaggerated fashion, doing the exercises with excessive energy and speed. Ms Ash had to slow her down and get her to start over again and explicitly told her to forget that she had ever been a physiotherapist.

Fourth meeting — Wednesday, 22nd March, 1972

Case 6 (Ms Ash) — follow-up
Firstly, an addendum to last week's discussion. Ms Ash wishes to emphasise that she felt misinterpreted by the seminar — ie seen as having been more crushing than she actually was to her physiotherapist-patient. She has seen her again and things are much as before. This report arose from somebody expressing disappointment about not having heard any miraculous follow-ups from the work of the seminar. The hope would be that a therapist had returned to the patient, armed with marvellously effective remarks that transform the situation.

110

Case 7 (Ms Ash)

Secondly, this week's case — cancer again. A slim attractive woman of 38 has had a mastectomy for cancer, very recently, is still having radiotherapy and is now referred for physiotherapy. She had an unexplained quarrel with the first physiotherapist and was transferred to Ms Ash by the department head. The patient asked Ms Ash whether she knew about the row and did she want to know about it? Ms Ash suggested it would be best if they tried to start off afresh. She examined the scar and admired it. Later the patient wanted to ask her about the diagnosis and prognosis, which Ms Ash evaded with the usual ploys of, 'What did your doctor say?' etc. The patient's father is also a doctor. Ms Ash had skilfully avoided acquiring any information about the prognosis and this was reflected in the seminar similarly avoiding this thorny point for half an hour. The policy is that it is better not to know. Nevertheless, they went on to discuss the effect on the patient, who obviously does know and wants to talk about it and yet is met with this sort of attitude.

There was quite a lot of discussion about what might have gone wrong with the previous physiotherapist. One impression was that it was to do with being treated 'in the gymn' — in a large room together with other patients, mainly neurological patients, paraplegics, etc. The problem hovers between anxiety about seeing other mutilated people versus anxiety about being exposed and mutilated oneself. Ms Ash conveyed the impression that she had struck a right note in making some attempt to tackle this latter angle by beginning with an inspection of the scar. She was willing to have a look but she was evidently not willing (and probably rightly so) to look at the 'scar' of the row with her predecessor. The seminar scrupulously avoided any investigation of Ms Ash's views of this predecessor and it was all left covered over by hopeful or vague sentiments that the row would probably have happened whoever it had been.

Following some themes about these difficulties and the time required to work through various aspects of it all, Ms Ash spelled out the way she felt it[1] was like teaching children at school. The most important things were those that could not be put into the text-books. You could only learn by experience. Ostensibly, I suppose she was talking about the wider problems of teaching but I pointed out the ambiguity and my impression that this was a reference to sexuality. However much the children may be taught and told, or given the facts of life etc, there is this childhood fact that you can't really know until you have experienced adulthood yourself, until you have been a mummy or daddy . . . I pointed out the clear awareness[2] of sexuality in all this together with feelings about the mutilation of a young woman and the feeling of helplessness to deal with it all. This accentuates the feeling that the scar might burst open.

This discussion sprang from some feeling in the seminar that the surgeons are *irrationally* afraid of physiotherapy for these patients. It is not explicit, but some of them are uneasy that physiotherapy will rock the boat — maybe causing the scar to burst open, fluid to accumulate underneath, or spread the cancer through all this violent movement pictured. But I went on to clarify my impression that this was not soley the anxiety of the surgeon.

Case 8 (Ms Elder)

She has conveyed an impression of quiet scepticism, due perhaps to being somewhat solemn-faced. Her actual comments are reasonably open-minded. She does tend to present herself as not having cases and therefore not having problems. This one was 'not really her case' because it was her student's case and anyway the patient had been referred to another surgical team on a day she was not there. In general, she emphasised, she is a member of an excellent team with good co-operation between surgeon, social worker, physiotherapist and all.

The patient is a woman in her 70s awaiting an operation (tibial osteotomy) for advanced rheumatoid-arthritis and osteo-arthritis. The houseman noticed a small lump in the breast which is cancer and the problem is what to do. Everybody is clear that it should come out but they cannot convey this to the patient who is dim and possibly a little deaf. Of course, it turns out that their failure to make the matter clear to this patient is compounded by their difficulty in making it clear to anybody else. Nobody uses the word cancer and nobody is willing to spell out what they are talking about, even without using the word cancer. What does the physiotherapist do *in her team* in such a case? We note that the matter has been left for the social worker 'to talk to the patient'. This makes sense so far as the social worker is the one most used to 'doing the talking'. But it makes very little sense in so far as the social worker is the person least equipped to talk about the dangers and indications and results of the various operations which are projected.

Notes
1 'It' being the problem of what to explain or disclose and how to put it.
2 The point here is that I am referring to *their* awareness and this is not a case of the psychoanalyst offering his peculiar interpretations.

Fifth meeting — Tuesday, 28th March, 1972

Case 9 (Ms Elm)
A man of 52, who looks 70, fell while drunk at New Year and had a Colles's fracture.[1] He was left with a tremendous amount of residual stiffness and pain and has been attending physiotherapy ever since — latterly daily. He is tremulous and terrified, making hardly any progress whatever they do. Ms Elm finds it very difficult to assess but clearly thinks that most of the trouble is mental. He is a postman and is now unable to work but has not yet lost his job. He is solitary, lives in a slum and has to carry his slops up and down stairs in a bucket. His only conviviality is in the pub where he appears to go every night — and in the physiotherapy department where he now comes every day. He is certainly portrayed as an isolated miserable man with an impoverished life but then this somehow seems very hard to admit as an explicit statement.

The seminar discussed various angles regarding the management of his treatment, eg trying him in groups or trying him with exercises that will simulate his work etc. Pain-relieving ice packs produced quite a bit of relief but no real progress. It emerges that he has been treated by a succession of students of variable calibre, and has now just lost a particularly good one. He burst into tears the other morning in the department and this seems to have put the lid on things. Ms Elm did then refer him back to the orthopaedic surgeon and received a written note stating, 'should progress'.

The discussion reflected closely the isolation of the patient and the seminar seemed to feel that the physiotherapist, too, is a totally isolated agent, who has to carry the world on her back. There seemed to be no idea of devising a more appropriate management for this man's miseries, now located in his wrist by mutual agreement, than pursuing physiotherapy. There is no sense of there being any colleagues to whom he might be referred and, when colleagues are discussed, it is as if they are on another planet, eg the Medical Officer of Health for the Borough is proposed. We also think of the Housing Department. Ms Elm seems to find enormous difficulty in confronting this man with his need for another treatment and, at any rate, the need to see the social worker, as a first step towards diagnosis. The GP might also be contacted. We note the contrast between the willingness to jolly the patient along through painful procedures against the unwillingness to put him through pain which will embarrass the therapist.

Case 10 (Ms Sycamore)
A lady of 74, hitherto working in a factory canteen, has a fracture of the neck of humerus and lower end of radius. The wrist is reasonable but the shoulder makes no progress. Ms Sycamore has taken over the treatment from her students and the problem she raises is why she has to put such an enormous amount of energy into the treatment of this patient. She feels that she has to push and push to get anywhere and can't understand what this is about and feels it to be wrong.

The patient squeaks and groans and clearly enjoys the idea of being subjected to a cruel treatment, with remarks like, 'You're not going to make me do it again are you?', 'You're going to be cruel again I can see . . . !' We observe but can't do much, on this occasion, with the observation that cruel treatment and love of the patient seem curiously fused at times. There was some discussion of the sense that this is an elderly lady and it might be reasonable not to push so much and not to expect such a good result. The seminar hide behind this to deny the anxieties about age and incurability. The question, 'Why don't you relax and let it go since she is old? Let her go away and be happy', contains and conceals the source of anxiety that is shared with the patient.[2] The fact is that the patient has been determined to resist old age by working hard at 74. I also felt that there was a retreat from the whole question of the meaning of the accident, from the question of how it happened, which was never asked, except by me. In order to suppress this issue they also had to suppress the professional physiotherapy question that should otherwise have arisen, viz how did this peculiar combination of fractures occur? Actually, it occurred through a fall downstairs but this does not really tell us all about it. We had to leave the discussion there.

Discussion
The plenary discussion was very lively and nearly everybody took part. Clearly the seminar aroused interest and some good-natured envy. The suggestion about the GP regarding the first case was salvaged in this discussion – it was a point we missed at first. This underlies the question of isolation as a real problem going right through the case. Other questions raised were whether we had talked much about job satisfaction for physiotherapists. Did Dr Bourne think, as was one impression, that physiotherapists are poor communicators? I tried to elaborate the feeling of needing time to work properly at the sort of issues raised, comparing and contrasting this time-scale with the time-scale prevailing in physiotherapy work itself. Again, the question of, 'Did you make progress?' carries another message about the spirit in which the work proceeds. I made the point that a lot of physiotherapy work does *not* go on in a climate of

hopeful expectation of progress or rather that this can never be admitted. It is clear that they carry an enormous burden of chronic illness but the notion that a patient may *need* to get worse[3] is heresy for them. This is at the centre of Ms Elm's case for example (actually of both).

Notes
1 Fracture of the radius at the wrist.
2 In other words, it does not squarely face the true possibility that it is a case of, 'Let her go away and be miserable'.
3 ie get more miserable.

Sixth meeting – Thursday, 25th May, 1972

Case 11 (Ms Oak)

A 48-year-old Spanish-Gibraltar woman, bedridden with disseminated sclerosis and flexion contractures. The houseman, nursing staff, etc, come and go and Ms Oak has been representing continuity for three-and-a-half years. She does not know how to cope with the alternating idealisation and denigration from this woman – mainly the latter. The consultant is maintained as an idealised receiver of smiles and conversation about the flowers on his weekly round. Everybody else comes in for the ups and downs, but especially Ms Oak. Others are the nurses, the occupational therapists, the medical social worker, etc.

We begin to see clearly that Ms Oak feels very maternal, as a result of being the only person who really has a continuous view of this patient. She has to hold herself back from constantly prompting and instigating the attentions that she thinks the patient requires, eg that she should be out in the sun, away on holiday, or is in danger of getting a bedsore if something is not done about the present position . . . Ms Mahogany expressed the sense that Ms Oak appears to be getting over-involved but, in the main, we get an impression of a fairly appropriate and understandable concern and that her observations and interfering impulses are largely appropriate. She and the patient are somewhat forced into this relationship with each other, although neither of them is really aware of it. Ms Oak is aware of being compared (usually adversely) with the English (she is foreign), the previous physiotherapist superintendent, etc but does not twig that she is basically being compared with the patient's mother. Gradually I felt very clear about the tense ambivalence both are feeling. The wish to send the patient out into the sun or away on holiday is transparently mingled with the wish to see her dead and get the bed empty. And death is the only solution to this case anyway. On the patient's side, Ms Oak, as 'mother', is the only person who 'really' cares and looks after her and is thereby simultaneously the persecutory object responsible for all her woes. Mostly, Ms Oak is the bad mother in order that the ward sister may be maintained as the idealised good mother. I was very interested in the way Ms Oak is simultaneously (a) the stranger, the foreigner, the woman with the foreign accent – very much the stranger of whom the baby is shy, terrified and (b) the most intimate of all people, the baby's mother – even down to having almost the same name (which I did not discuss). The patient has complained of her as being foreign. I tried to draw attention and interest towards this question of the fear of strangers, the sort of primitive paranoid anxiety that every medical and paramedical person encounters, especially with new patients, but also with old ones all the time. It seems obvious and automatic that something strange and foreign should be frightening but I reminded them that, in its pure form, we see this as a special feature of a certain phase of development in babies.

Seventh meeting – Wednesday, 8th June, 1972

Case 3 (Ms Sycamore) – follow-up

A woman in her 50s with breast cancer or cancer phobia. We had previously discussed this patient but all managed to forget that there had been a mastectomy 20 years ago and Ms Sycamore did not remind us until recapitulating the case for a newcomer. The patient previously had been nagging the physiotherapist as to what the doctor thought and the physiotherapist was pushed into evasion. Previously the physiotherapy was given in connection with a pathological fracture of the hip and the referral was then from the radiotherapy department.

Since then she has fallen and fractured her shoulder and is now referred by the orthopaedic surgeon. It seems that *he* told the patient that she *did* have a tumour of the spine which was dealt with by the radiotherapy.

For whatever reason, there is much less nagging and Ms Sycamore is really raising the issue of why the improvement? The mystery is whether the patient is better, (a) because somebody has been more honest or, (b) because somebody has been successfully reassuring. Linked with either of these possibilities is a plan to go to Lourdes this autumn. It seems, also, that the social worker has been active and the patient has been equipped with a mobile chair suitable to go into the car. Unfortunately her husband has a cataract and cannot drive at the moment.

We still get a sense of Ms Sycamore not daring to go an inch further than the way the doctor has set it up – but yet unable really to clarify with the doctor as to how he *has* set it up.

Case 12 (Ms Elm)

A man of 48 with rheumatoid arthritis. He is a keen amateur wrestler – latterly involved with training more than wrestling himself. He is also a docker. The rheumatoid arthritis was of sudden severe onset and we are told it carries a bad prognosis. The physical medicine doctor, referring the patient, did confer with Ms Elm (he is very good about this) and said that he had spelt it out to the patient who had clearly refused to grasp it. Ms Elm was specifically charged with helping him to grasp it.

The patient is a very polite, nicely-dressed man who's always immaculately turned out and brings his own gym shorts, declining to use the department's ones. He is angry and complaining about the failure to progress. He asks for something stronger than the aspirins he is now given. He refuses to make any alteration in his plans or outlook regarding work and Ms Elm is at a loss to know how to get him to change his attitude.

Actually he is not 'having treatment' at the moment and she merely passes him from time to time as he sits waiting his turn in the out-patient department. This raises the question of how much it is a part of the physiotherapist's work to 'be around' the department in order to keep tabs on patients and to be in touch with colleagues. (This is painfully with us since Ms Ash will probably have to leave the seminar as she may be required to be in a clinic which has been moved to Thursday afternoons.)

We gradually delineate Ms Elm's inability to get into the case, in the sense of recognising him in particular, rather than the problem in general. She

115

announces but then ignores the fact that he is interested in wrestling. How important is this and in what way? We also get a sense of her isolation and the patient's isolation. In spite of the discussion with the doctor there is only a precarious sense of working in any convincing sense *with* colleagues. Only belatedly does the question of occupational therapy come in. The patient is pictured as totally isolated and somebody wonders whether he would be able to open tins -- as if he lives alone and does for himself. He does have a family but Ms Elm never sees them. Why not? Where are they?

Eighth meeting -- Thursday, 15th June, 1972

Case 13 (Ms Poplar)

An Italian aged 32. An ex-athlete who was injured, paraplegic, by a British bullet in Aden, was brought to England for treatment and has remained. He has some family here, mainly an uncle and aunt and their daughter, a doctor at X Hospital.

He has a moderately severe paraplegia but can walk with crutches. The injury occurred when he was 19 (he is now about 32). A few years ago he developed cervical myelopathy (? due to virus) with severe residual wasting and loss of movement in the hands. His arms remain powerful.

He is a handsome, charming young man but it is only after prolonged discussion and underlining from me that his sexual presence is acknowledged openly. The problem presented is that he has severe attacks of screaming when he arrives in the physiotherapy department and, occasionally, at other times. Ms Poplar has the impression of some psychological basis to this, eg he screams when he loses at poker but not when he is winning! She thinks he screams when she confronts him with difficult exercises. The feeling appears to be that no physical explanation is available to explain these attacks of pain.

Meanwhile, he has been on regular doses of analgaesics but there is a bit of a mystery here -- some story of injections of codeine phosphate and a plan, begun yesterday, to replace them by sterile water. All very peculiar. I felt that this rather weird treatment reflects a weird picture of this man and perhaps it is to do with some picture of his damaged sexuality. There was some mention of possible programmes of work (sic) in relation to an awareness of this problem for paraplegics. Not exactly their sexual rehabilitation but something.

He has been in a succession of hospitals, often discharged after only a few days. He causes great disturbance to staff and other patients and has been known to hit staff over the head with his crutch.

Ms Poplar kept comparing the pains to labour pains and I took this to be a reference to some sense of the underlying passion, ie that this is not merely to be explained as a general expression of misery bursting out, although there is plenty of that. I also felt that the way she kept tying herself up on the word 'emasculate' or 'emasculinate' (together with the labour pains idea) referred to a sense of the confusion about his sexuality. I thought that all this disturbed the staff handling him and interfered with what little it might be possible to do.

A final point -- she mentioned that he pushed his chair out onto the roof and the hospital is slap in the middle of a red-light area where he is subjected to the disturbance of all the sexual goings-on in the street there and the pornographic bookshop opposite. I added that this might disturb the staff too.

Case 11 (Ms Oak) – follow-up
On Anna the lady from Gibraltar. A new locum houseman (female) tackled Ms Oak a day or two ago, having been told of some imagined atrocity by Anna. The others felt Ms Oak should be very angry and indignant but Ms Poplar insisted that there were patient-beaters around and that it was the doctors' duty to take such an accusation seriously. There was some brief discussion of the attitude towards, and handling of, the doctor.

Ms Oak had kept away from the patient in the hope of avoiding this but may have got the interval wrong: and all the bitter complaint may reflect the patient's need for her and anxiety about losing her. Ms Poplar was very explicit about this and kept making parallels between a mother and her little boy.

Ninth meeting – Thursday, 22nd June, 1972

Case 11 (Ms Oak) – follow-up
Ms Oak reported her latest encounter with Anna in which she had been able to suppress many of her previous annoyances and allowed Anna to hold her hand, in a state of pleasant affection.

Case 14 (Ms Oak)
Another case of a woman aged about 60, who probably has had disseminated sclerosis for many years, undiagnosed until a recent accident produced severe disability. The essence of the case is the patient's unexpected ability to walk 'for the consultant' and, infuriatingly, inability to do anything much 'for Ms Oak', a day or two later. She says that, with the seminar in mind, she was able to keep her temper. Instead, she was able to extricate the patient from the fantasy of doing it for the doctor and not doing it for the physiotherapist, and to draw attention to the realities about doing it in the service of her own future. Ms Oak pointed out that, 'you are too young to spend the rest of your life in a chair'. This is all very well and sounds quite successful but actually Ms Oak does not go in for losing her temper and it is tricky to know what, if any, influence the seminar did have.[1] Ms Poplar also pointed out the fact that Ms Oak does seem to have a knack of succeeding with these patients – a comment with undercurrents of suspicion. ('You don't actually bring *problems*, do you?')

Case 15 (Ms Ash)
This was about the handling of a blind colleague, a youngster working in the department of which she is head.[2] This girl is very selfish and demanding, resents doing her share of any chores and always wants to push in first with her patients, keeping everybody else waiting. Of course, this is very difficult and nobody likes to be hard on her as she is blind. However, there is a clear feeling that the difficulty has little immediately to do with her blindness but is a defect of her personality. Ms Ash also remarked that the girl is unusually attached to her father. Recently Ms Ash lost her temper and ticked her off, resulting in some improvement, but she feels very uncomfortable about it.[3]

This led to some delicate recognition of the fact that there is more than one type of blindness and that some of these personality problems are not confined to blind colleagues. Actually, as the seminar were arriving today, I was on the phone to a member of their organisation to discuss official recognition of the seminar as 'a course'. This had led to some snide remarks about the lack of co-operation you can expect from 'them', but behind this, the question of what sort of preference you could expect from colleagues.

Case 6 (Ms Ash) — follow-up
On the patient who was also a physiotherapist, described during our first few weeks. Ms Ash was still in some confusion about how to handle this woman and how far to recognise or blind herself to the fact that she is a physiotherapist — or was one at any rate.

Notes
1 The tape-recording of this session makes matters much clearer. Ms Oak realised that the patient's behaviour was calculated to enlist the doctor's support for an apparently successful treatment and then to force Ms Oak to work all the harder at it. Ms Oak then showed the patient that it was better to walk than to remain attached to a devoted physiotherapist.
2 She herself is well under 30.
3 There was resentment at the succession of patients who kept saying, 'Isn't she marvellous!'

Tenth meeting — Thursday, 29th June, 1972

Case 13 (Ms Poplar) — follow-up
The Italian athlete who screams. The situation has developed into a battle of love-hate between Ms Poplar and the patient. She had decided to push him harder than ever, forcing him to walk and he, in turn, is screaming more and more, with daily attacks of vomiting, which she has to clean up. It also re-emerges that he is being shifted to Stoke Mandeville[1] in a couple of weeks.

I was struck by their capacity to recognise all sorts of things about the situation and yet the inability to connect it with the screaming. It was noticed that he probably has mixed feelings about going to Stoke Mandeville — high hopes but also considerable fear. He is repeatedly sent from one place to the other and can never settle anywhere. There is all the untouched sexual excitement recognised in overt flirtation. There is the anger stirred in the therapist ('but I'm not going to let him see that he upsets me'). There is the distress of being so disabled. Ms Popular maintains that he has done his worst and there is nothing he can do now to make things worse — which is swiftly recognised as gross denial by the others. When this is exposed we find frank fears in Ms Poplar that he will give himself cardiac arrest or God knows what else.

But the point is that nobody can make the step to say that he may be screaming because he is angry, because he is afraid, because he is miserable, because he is excited . . . as the case may be. Ms Poplar's hunches would take her in the direction of trying to discuss his anger, so this may be the central problem but there are the other possibilities. It is clearly recognised that there is a sort of collusive contract that the only parley between them may be flirtatious chats about wine, food and sunshine. Apart from the screaming, he always has to be smiling and making eyes. They feel quite fixed on the single notion of asking him why he is screaming and being told either that he does not know or that it is because of the pain. No physiotherapist feels licensed to make an empathic remark, let alone an interpretation.

118

Case 16 (Ms Mahogany)

Another patient who is always moaning and miserable and disliked by all the staff and all the other patients in the ward. He is a West Indian and is suspected of being a homosexual. The seminar skirt around a discussion of everybody else's obvious prejudices and then admit their own too, reasonably honestly. I wondered how far the sense of this patient as a weird persecuting object, hated and feared, is possibly related to his illness too. There is a story, which I missed turning over the tape; he had a thoracotomy a few months ago and a cardiac biopsy — so obscure was his diagnosis at that point. I think he presented with multiple joint swellings and was evidently very ill. The diagnosis of miliary tuberculosis has been reached. He is now beginning to improve quite a bit and should continue to mend. But he is hard to get on his feet and to get moving.

I thought there was a denial of the effect upon staff of these patients with mysterious diagnoses who take a long time to get better. Also, was there no phobia of tuberculosis itself? This thought was stirred by a discussion about whether masks were worn in treating him — the point being raised that they might make him feel an inferior outcast and therefore paranoid. What is side-stepped is the professional staff's actual fear of catching something from him. Some members admitted readily they would be afraid, others denied it.[2]

Case 17 (Ms Sycamore)

The problem of a junior colleague. She emphasised that these personality problems are more troublesome amongst subordinates than in peers. We hear that this student tends to be sharp and tactless with the patients and that her attempts to jolly them along, in the traditional physiotherapist's manner, turn into something rather acid. There the discussion flies off into the possible handling of all sorts of imaginary difficulties that other students might exhibit — and thence to the syndrome of giving a dog a bad name and another syndrome of students who are blacklisted for wearing lipstick etc by old-fashioned tutors. It had been mentioned that this girl has taken years extra through repeatedly failing exams all the way along. There is actually no suggestion at all that her problem has anything to do with using lipstick.

We did not get any further with a specific elucidation of how she does annoy people and I suggested that perhaps our main concern at the moment was to do with feelings about subordinates, inferiors, potential victims, that we feel inclined to attack. Ms Elm last week mentioned what a nightmare it was to be an examiner, struggling against the temptation 'to sink people'. Strangely enough the only chapter and verse we did then get was of an episode in which Ms Sycamore's offending student had placed a very small woman patient in the pool, with the water up over her nose. Everybody had been down on her very quickly for this. We had to stop at the end, in the middle of a discussion about preparing students for examinations. I was struck by the flavour of people feeling they had to rig the situation, in order to 'make a point' in relation to their students,[3] rather than having any sense that people could be more genuinely helped towards their final examination.

Notes

1 Stoke Mandeville Hospital — a nationally famous centre for the treatment of paraplegics and spinal injuries.
2 The fear of 'catching something' from patients might be supposed to be

obvious and even banal. Actually there is a taboo on such 'cowardly' anxieties with the result that appropriate precautions are often neglected.

3 As teachers, they develop a repertoire of ruses and ploys and there is a constant sense of them trying to help their students through an obstacle race, formed by the caprices or prejudices of senior members of the profession.

Eleventh meeting – Thursday, 6th July, 1972

Case 18 (Ms Elm)

This occupied most of the time. A porter from Covent Garden was said to have had a 20 lb package fall on his neck, but with no perceptible injury. He arrived in the physiotherapy department with an orthopaedic collar and himself hunched down into it. It is impossible to get him to move anything and he complains of pain on being asked to make almost any movement anywhere. He is supposed to attend daily but disappeared for a couple of weeks. Ms Elm was short with him on his return and he crumpled abjectly, having been rather belligerent until this time. She then felt sorry for having been hard on him. There are then further hints to Ms Elm herself and the senior student who shares his treatment with her – hints of his wife's depression and how she is constantly away on holiday, eg six months in Malta last year. There appears to be some willingness to tackle the possible compensation neurosis angle, if that is what it is all about, although even this seems to be rather prickly. What is impossible is to take up any of his offers to talk about his marriage and about himself. The difficulty in taking these things up is understandable and quite possibly appropriate but what is more interesting is the difficulty for the physiotherapists here to be honest with themselves. It is difficult for them to spell out to themselves their firm diagnosis – based on careful accumulated observation – that there is no physical condition to treat, except possibly some muscular spasm.

At one point in the discussion the possible referral to a medical social worker was raised. Joking swiftly revealed the underlying sense of this man's possible 'need for a floozie', ie their fear of occupying this sort of role. It is hard to know whether the physiotherapist feels more like a floozie or less like one, if she is honest with herself about the nature of the case she is treating and the nature of what she is doing. There is some clamour about the possibility of being honest and open about sexuality with patients upon whom you are laying hands. This appeared, in the discussion, to take in completely the difficulty about being honest with oneself too. Is it all right to provide quack remedies, physical gratifications etc, if one is not licensed by some shred of doubt leaving open the possibility that 'it is really physical'?

It is also evident that this man is seen as probably impotent and yet this thought could only reach the light of day after much work in the seminar. Ms Poplar said it was the first thing she thought but did not feel that the climate of the seminar would allow her to say so.

Case 13 (Ms Poplar) – follow-up

Her Italian man, the athlete. She reports a bald-headed bull-at-a-gate attempt to tackle him with questions. 'Are you worried about the future? Are you worried about leaving for Stoke Mandeville?' She received a flat denial on all these points. I was surprised that she was surprised but we did not particularly discuss this. One point of interest was her mention that he had attempted to head a football. It landed on his boil, which must have been extremely painful, yet his response was one of normal pain, stoically met, in contrast to the other carry-on.

Case 16 (Ms Mahogany) – follow-up
Her West Indian patient. It seems he has become more ill and everybody has become more sympathetic towards him. He, in turn, has become more co-operative and tries harder with his treatment. It is hard to know at which point in the cycle change was initiated. No mention was made of the possibility that she may have initiated some change, although she did repeat that throughout she had remained more benign towards him than everybody else.

Case 19 (Ms Sycamore)
'Old Mr Carter'. Heard only in the last quarter hour. A 74-year-old man with an above-knee amputation. He also has chronic bronchitis and recent congestive heart failure. Ms Sycamore has to get him mobilised. His son says he has always been disagreeable and he certainly is now – very unpleasant to everybody, boorish and alienating. He has 10 or 11 children. His wife is said to be an invalid and he is very worried about her too. How on earth are they going to manage? Of all the children, it seems that only one daughter will help look after them and she is being paid for the purpose. This is generally felt to reflect his unlovableness. The problem is that he is very hard to get doing anything and complains of being messed around all the time. Eventually he exasperated Ms Sycamore until she said, 'No! You are messing us about!' The ward staff had tried to cajole and exhort him with such pleasant remarks as, 'You don't want to have to go to a home, do you'. To this he replies that he does, and insists that his picture of a home is of a sort of Eden where everything will be done for him.

There was an interesting little exchange about his going to Roehampton (regional centre for artificial limbs) for an artificial limb to be fitted. For whatever reason, this proved to be impossible and he said something about having 'had to have the mask on' while he was there. This referred to some sort of collapse requiring oxygen. Ms Elm responded with a half-jocular free-association, taking him to mean that he had to wear a mask because the other patients were smelly. Behind this I had a sense of the way amputees are seen as smelly bits of shit and that this is the feeling about him as somebody who is going to lose his other leg and die pretty soon. This is the way he sees himself and probably the way the staff see him too. I felt that the staff involved have great difficulty in controlling the mixture of hatred and contempt which he arouses and which, they feel, ought not to be there: they ought of course to feel concern, compassion, respect, etc. I did mention my sense of this problem of contempt and linked it with Ms Elm's case where the feelings of contempt for the impotent man were more obvious.

Right at the end there was a little discussion about the daft facetious ideas they use to get these people going. 'We'll put you in for the Derby/the Oaks etc!' 'They could do with you for Chelsea!' 'We'll have you in next year's Olympics', etc. Ms Poplar closed the session by reporting how one such piece of levity on her part, a few days ago, was answered by the old man telling her to piss off.

Twelfth meeting — Thursday, 13th July, 1972

Case 13 (Ms Poplar) — follow-up

Described as 'a real blow in the solar plexus'. Franco, the Italian athlete, was given infra-red treatment for his back while Ms Poplar was away on holiday last week and has undergone a miraculous recovery from the screaming and vomiting attacks. It is open to speculation how far this miracle is connected with her holiday, how far connected with the sudden novelty of fresh interest by the house physician — extending even to a specific physiotherapy-type prescription of infra-red treatment. Just possibly, the suggestion came from Franco himself, who had once had infra-red treatment for a bedsore. It is also clear that he has not been pushed so much during Ms Poplar's absence but he has been able to do things that, in her hands, would have induced screaming.

I was surprised that they were not more interested in this intervention by the house physician into what would seem to me to be their territory. I also had a sense of this man, fallen amongst women, responding to a man's support. It is also of some interest that the prescription (for infra-red) arrived at the department verbally, via Franco himself, who simply said that he had been talking to the house physician and had been asked to bring down this suggestion. 'Presumably' it was checked over the phone.

Case 19 (Ms Sycamore) — follow-up

'Old Mr Carter', the above-knee amputee. The 'social work development' is really a move to send him home because the surgeons want the bed. She was not consulted and feels slighted. To this extent, she is inclined to sympathise and line up with the patient, who is otherwise completely alienating. He remains grumpy and complaining. She gave a fairly detailed account of his visit to the physiotherapy department this morning when he dissolved into tears, talking about the possibility of going home. The plan is that he goes home in a wheelchair and ostensibly, his main fear is of being a burden to his ill wife. I thought they picked up, but could not spell out, the sense he has of being a burden *to them*. The temptation is to connect this mainly with his present disability and bad prognosis although we have an uneasy awareness that he has always been a grumpy old man and has 11 children who do not want him. Ms Sycamore is able to confront him with his tiresomeness when she is sufficiently angry while at the same time actually working to help him, eg trying to make him walk. It seems much more difficult to acknowledge with him, in cold blood, that he is grumpy, objectionable and unwanted. Thus, his recurrent complaint, 'I don't know why they keep sending me down here', is an opening to spell out his awareness that they are sending him down because they do not want him upstairs.

We did not get very far with the question of how Ms Sycamore would behave regarding the ward staff who slight her — either forgetting about her or (more probably true for the nurses) actually wanting to exclude her. She murmured her intention of making sure to join the ward rounds in future, which struck me, interestingly, as being a less paranoid way of behaving than my own might have been. I said nothing of this.

Case 20 (Ms Poplar)

'Gorgeous Gussie'. An 'old woman' of 58, 'old enough' to have been in the ATS during the war. She has been attending the hospital since 1942, following post-encephalitic Parkinsonism. Latterly she has been coming with osteo-arthritic knees. The point really is that she is the pet of an 'old'

122

consultant – also in his 50s – a gentlemanly type, very courtly and polite to his patients, very correct in his black pinstripe suit. Nobody is ever discharged from that hospital – they always get a follow-up appointment until death. Now the hospital itself is threatened with closure and this may be what it is all about. However, the immediate problem is that she practically lives in the department, coming up five times a week and arriving hours before her appointment. No treatment is really effective. Gorgeous Gussie is a strange character who talks at Speakers' Corner in Hyde Park, keeps 'five cats who have dysentery over her bed when she is away' and so on.

There is a clear sense of a mixture of excitement, madness and cruelty. Ms Poplar quite frankly describes her plan of giving painful treatments that would induce her to go somewhere else but is quite surprised when this is recognised as cruelty or sadism by her colleagues. This must somewhere be relevant to the problem of excitement laced with sado-masochism in all her accounts. She mentions that she hates treating osteo-arthritis and went to work at this neurological hospital where her interest lies. (She also mentioned that her sister's tumour, presumably cerebral, renewed or turned her interest in this direction.) So there is all that behind it too.

Ms Sycamore said she would be quite interested to try treating this lady and I think she meant it. The patient is said to get £19 a week in various benefits, including her army pension. After the tape was switched off and time was up, further talk revealed that she wears out a pair of gym shoes each week and somehow gets the necessary money from 'the 'elp'. This seems also to be a bizarre and important angle which we could not quite get hold of.

Thirteenth meeting – Thursday, 20th July, 1972

Case 13 (Ms Poplar) – follow-up
Her Italian athlete. It is now more or less explicit that he screams and vomits when she treats him but not when treated by a less experienced colleague. This may be simply because she pushes him harder to attempt things, but it seems more likely that it is something personal, related to the intensity of their relationship. He appears to like her very much so it is certainly not a simple matter. The colleague is unable to attempt the things Ms Poplar does, unless she has somebody to assist her, and it is said that there is nobody and that an unskilled porter is not really good enough and not available anyway. I thought that there was something important about this question of being 'the one and only' as we seem to be involved with a syndrome of cases who are all the one and only. Each physiotherapist tends to bring one special case as her case, as if there is no other. Ms Poplar is evidently some sort of 'one and only' for this chap. Ostensibly, she is worried lest he go to Stoke Mandeville and is promptly bounced back again because he 'won't try'. The back pain, 'cured' by infra-red, (see last week) has not returned but he now screams with pain in the legs and says infra-red won't be any good.

Case 21 (Ms Mahogany)
A 23-year-old Canadian hotel telephonist dislocated her patella. She was anxious not to have it removed and was offered an operation that would stabilise it. On operation, it was found that the technique was not going to work and they proceeded to remove the patella. The problem is that she appears now to be totally incapable of getting her quadriceps going again.

A variety of plasters, splints, back-slabs and plastic supports have been employed and she is now being discharged to return for out-patient physiotherapy.

Ms Mahogany first encountered the patient last Saturday and gave her 20 minutes (apparently a long time). The patient is noisy and garrulous, very friendly, very admiring of English surgeons. It is known that her mother died a year or two ago and that she has a father in Canada to whom she is devoted and writes every day. Some scepticism arises about her having left him in this context.

It is recognised that keeping her patella had exaggerated meaning for her in the first place and that she must now be concealing strong unconscious feelings about what was done during the operation — 'removing her bits and bobs' (Ms Poplar, who also saw her as feeling violated under the anaesthetic).

The clinical problem is excessive pain and fear of the leg being unsupported. She will not even hang it down while sitting and she cannot be tricked into using the quads muscles by all the range of physiotherapy tricks they try out. I wondered about this business of tricks on a patient who must already be feeling tricked.

The elements were there in the discussion but I had to make the connection between this need to feel held and supported and some feelings about the dead mother. The seminar had already decided that they, the physiotherapists, were in turn correspondingly worried about the quadricps. They probably would get going anyway in somebody of that age and the spectre of them disappearing altogether does not have too much basis here. I said something about the anatomy of the family as compared with the anatomy of the thigh and said that they seem to have some feelings, shared with the patient, about these quads as being to do with the mother who holds you. This was received sceptically but led, as a free association, to Ms Elm's case which she brought up thereupon *en passant*. A handsome confirmation of the point in question.

Case 22 (Ms Sycamore)
A nurse has an operation on her knee owing to grindings and clickings. The knee joint is found to have a number of fibrous bands, cause unknown, which the surgeon cuts. Following her operation it is, as with Ms Mahogany's case, totally impossible to get the quads going. It was a brief report, but it is mentioned as a final afterthought, that *her mother is a physiotherapist*.

The point of the story is that suddenly, from one day to the next, all changed in a way which Ms Sycamore found almost impossible to believe. Suddenly the muscle changed from blancmange into a working unit and they have been very rapidly able to get on to heavy exercises. She has no idea what has caused the change, but it underlines the sense that some of the physiotherapist's anxieties about the disappearance of the quads have more basis in fantasy than in reality. I pointed out too that we were really being given confirmation of some sense of connection between (1) this muscle that holds the legs; (2) the physiotherapist and her work which must be felt to provide some reliable holding; and (3) the physiotherapist/mother of the patient.

Fourteenth meeting — Thursday, 27th July, 1972

Case 23 (Ms Oak)

The problem of discharging a lady of 81 from hospital. She has been in for some months for treatment of stress fractures of a leg. There was a setback with conjunctivitis a couple of weeks ago. Now she is recovered and ready for discharge but dissolves into tears whenever it is mentioned. Ms Oak is left, or feels left, with the task of getting her out of hospital. The consultant left this decision on his weekly ward round and it is not too clear how the decision is really made and who implements it. But she feels it is on her plate.

Patient lives in a flat above a pub run by her son and grand-daughter. Daughter's husband does not appear in the picture. Patient adores grand-daughter but there is no particular sign of her interest in the patient. The family seem friendly but really take minimal interest and never have time to undertake any errands, eg Ms Oak had herself to see about buying outdoor shoes — making the actual purchase: the family were willing to pay.

The patient says more or less openly, 'You are throwing me out'. Ms Oak is not able to get to grips with the problem nor able to decide who should. The social worker has been involved in making arrangements and probably should take over more of the problem, especially at the family end. Ms Oak is probably lost in her recurrent role of motherliness.

Case 24 (Ms Elm)

Presented at an early stage and she foresees more trouble. The referral arrives carrying his own card, stating: 'Cervical Spondylosis' with a big question mark after it and 'try traction'. The student treating him is reduced to helpless fury and Ms Elm soon finds why. When you attempt to get any history from this patient, he rambles into endless irrelevances and peculiarities. He does not strike her as mad but makes her wonder if she is herself going mad. He talks about his pain in the back as being tubular in the middle, circular on one side, conical on the other. He does not appear to understand or to absorb any instructions about his appointments and is, as above, impossible to discuss anything with. He is also very intrusive, has no hesitation in bursting into Ms Elm's conversations with others, will follow her down a corridor and stand at her elbow while she makes a private telephone call.

We are really left with our speculations and associations at this point. We have to think about the nature of the referral and his possible reactions to what he will have read on the card. He is a builder and it was suggested that he may be one of these 'tomorrow-for-certain-madam' builders. Is he getting a tomorrow-for-certain-madam type of treatment with no real diagnosis, prognosis, or plan? Is Ms Elm, without realising it, caught up in a role which forces her to talk to him just as obscurely as he talks to her?

Case 25 (Ms Poplar)

This is raised as an example of a general problem — the person whose cervical collar never fits, like the person whose dentures never fit. This is an Andy Capp type of patient who refers to her as 'that girl'. She appears to have a good relationship, with good mutual esteem, between her and the neurologist consultant but this chap has managed to establish with the consultant the conviction that she is unable to fit a collar. She has given this chap every collar in the book, has referred him to X Hospital (another department), but still the collar never fits.

The tactics of handling this sort of patient will have to be explored but we are also involved with some sort of over-investment by Ms Poplar too. As part of a package to get senior grading, she had to accept the post of surgical appliances supplier and there is an amusing situation in that there is no superior person to be invoked. I drew attention to a sense that something unpleasant between consultant and physiotherapist may be canalised into something like this, leaving the rest of their relationship apparently more free of it. The patient requires the collar for cervical spondylosis, with the development of some spasticity in the legs, so that it is essential.

The problems of this case are intertwined with one of our other recurring motifs – the position of the poor struggling woman in a man's world. Are the Andy Capp patient and elderly male consultant in league to belittle 'that girl'?

Fifteenth meeting – 6th September, 1972

Case 23 (Ms Oak) – follow-up
She reported that 'Anna' is still there just the same, but we also had a follow-up of her other case of the old lady who lived over the pub. It now emerges that there was a blindness or wishful thinking in the entire staff group that made them see her as a member of a united family with loving granddaughter etc and a mystery as to why she would not go home. A more open-eyed exposure to a family meeting left the medical social worker in tears and Ms Oak providing cups of tea afterwards. Following this episode – and whatever the connection – the patient was able to make a trial visit home and then be discharged from hospital a few days later. Patient's tears and angry protests about being pushed out seem to have stopped. Is this an episode in which the new ability of the staff to 'have a problem' enabled some progress to be made in the handling of the case?

Case 19 (Ms Sycamore) – follow-up
The leg amputee in his 70s. She has given up the battle. The picture now changes to some recognition of the impending death of this man of 74 with one leg amputated for artereosclerosis and the other leg already developing ulcers. He has a bad heart, has had a stroke in the past . . . Ms Sycamore does not know whether to feel bad about having given up the struggle but the effect is now that he is placid and good-natured, whereas before he was evil-tempered and persecuted. She also mentioned that he had developed some difficulty with his anal sphincter, so that there was faecal dripping when they did get him standing up and this really put the finishing touch. It was recognised that the physiotherapist had to accept a wound to her pride (and omnipotence) to arrive at this reasonable adaptation.

Case 4 (Ms Elm) – follow-up
On her first case in the seminar (see session 8th March, 1972) – the man she had tried to discharge but who quickly got his word in first to the orthopaedic surgeon. She ran across him as she walked through the out-patient department and was astonished to be roundly abused. He appears to have had a fifth arthroplasty (three on one hip, two on the other) but had not been referred for physiotherapy this time. He was 'surprised that you

126

haven't been sacked yet . . . ' Although things had been cool before, she was shocked and hurt to get this mouthful.

Case 13 (Ms Poplar) – follow-up
The Italian athlete. After letting things drift for five weeks in the hands of her junior she was forced (she felt) to intervene again to get him going. The cycle instantly renewed itself with shrieking and puking etc. She took a stand in what is beginning to emerge as a battle with the rest of the hospital and got a psychiatric referral, with great difficulty. The result, predictably, was the 'diagnosis' that he 'did not seem to be depressed' but that 'a drug Dr X always prescribes' could be tried.

Following all this I brought up my impression that much of the discussion was about rows and battles with patients which were muddled up with battles between the professions and staff groups. From this it emerged that Ms Elm has given notice at her hospital, having allowed herself to recognise the depths of her dissatisfaction with the place and with orthopaedic surgeons whose work she suspects. She is going to another hospital in a month or so. It only emerged at the end that this threatens to prevent her coming on Wednesdays. We will know later.

Case 26 (Ms Poplar)
She wanted to raise the general question of her hospital's impending closure and what should she tell patients, but I induced her to raise a specific case. She chose a woman with disseminated sclerosis and her fears or doubts about transferring her to the X Hospital. She already comes a long way, from Acton, and the X Hospital really is just as near. We very swiftly got back to Ms Poplar's battle with the hospital and the NHS. She too colludes with the mystery-mongering – not only by refusing to find out properly what will happen (as far as this can be done) but by colluding in a cloak and dagger atmosphere. She laughingly describes how she steamed open a consultant's letter in order to get some information about the closing date. This appears to be some time in October. Her own professional future is in difficulty over this, since she requires a part-time senior or superintendent job in central London if she is not to be worse off. She lives in Greenwich and X Hospital is too far to go. A further complication – she prefers that the work be in a particular field of medicine (this has previously been mentioned as connected with her feelings about her twin sister's illness).

Returning to the patient, all this carried implications of what the patient's own anxieties and difficulties might be, how far they are linked with attachment to Ms Poplar herself as distinct from other aspects such as her attachment to the consultant, the hospital, the routine, etc. Behind this would be further questions about her clinical prognosis. All suggestions from the physiotherapists were to indicate possible lines of reassurance and 'management' and I had to face them with all this as being a clear alternative to the line in which the patients are faced not with reassurance but recognition of their anxiety. All this of course going back to the initial problem of looking for problems versus looking for successes.

Sixteenth meeting – 13th September, 1972

Case 27 (Ms Oak)
The central point here is something of a row with the ward sister, which has never happened before. An elderly patient is due for discharge and needs

more physiotherapy as an out-patient. On the other hand, she is quite incapable of coping without a great deal of support. She will need to spend long periods of each day in the physiotherapy department and this entails problems of care that they cannot cope with. There are enormous difficulties about procuring meals, as well as attending to the toilet needs of the patient.

All this might be part of an obvious and generally recurrent type of problem but in this case there seem to be two distinctive features. One is that Ms Oak was rather pushed and, against her better judgement, came up to speak to the sister about it just before lunchtime. There are suspicions that both she and the sister might have been suffering from low blood sugars and feelings of quite an infantile kind, while waiting for lunch. The second point is that a new day hospital type of unit is about to open in two or three weeks and this will be the obvious answer for this patient and others like her. It is set up to cope with exactly this sort of problem. Again, like the baby waiting for his feed, there is a feeling of exaggerated impatience and excitement as the time draws near. The excitement is not only over lovely new feeding facilities but also lovely new lavatories ... This hitches onto interprofessional rivalries, including the nurses' suspicion that a physiotherapist would not demean herself to carry a bed pan.

Seventeenth meeting – Wednesday, 20th September, 1972

Case 28 (Ms Mahogany)

A woman of 35 with rheumatoid arthritis. It is a chronic case admitted for treatment of severe contractures, fixing hips and knees in the flexed position. She was admitted for three weeks of bed-rest. Halfway through, Ms Mahogany returned from a course at Cambridge, fired with enthusiasm to try out a new regime of very active treatment in splints, under cover of heavy analgaesic doses. The proper regime requires a number of weeks but the doctors gave Ms Mahogany sanction to try for the remaining week of this woman's stay.

She rapidly discovered that in spite of very careful explanation of the procedures and the apparent understanding and agreement of the patient, she was actually getting no co-operation. The woman never did her exercises except when supervised. She did not spend any time lying in the prescribed positions – and, indeed, spent most of the time in positions that Ms Mahogany had forbidden! She also complained that she was not getting her analgaesics, was not sleeping and was 'really rather pathetic'.

The ward sister and another colleague, of whom Ms Mahogany holds high opinions, confirm their experience of various difficulties with this patient. The ward sister says she is rather odd and there is a story of her having three children of her own but that there was a fourth illegitimate baby given into adoption a couple of years ago. We do not know the source of this information nor what to do with it. Ms Mahogany has tried to discuss her home life with the patient, but gets absolutely nowhere.

Firstly, the seminar wonder about the bearing of Ms Mahogany's enthusiasm for the treatment on the present situation. Does Ms Mahogany's enthusiasm for a new treatment fail to give the patient a sense of any enthusiasm for the patient herself? However, usual experience is that staff enthusiasms for new treatments tend to be infectious and the sheer novelty of any new treatment usually brings some success. The point we have to grasp here is that this patient may have a strong pressure to remain disabled and that *this* is what brings her into collision with Ms Mahogany's enthusiasm for a new treatment.

We return to the mystery of the woman herself but cannot get any further. She was previously being treated at X Hospital and asked to be referred to Ms Mahogany's hospital, having heard of the specialist there. What now comes over to us is the extreme difficulty in seeing her in the context of her own background. It is possible that this admission to a hospital some distance from home has something to do with a specific wish or need on the patient's part to dislocate herself from home. 'Admission for bed rest' is, when you come to think about it, rather transparently little more than a move to 'get away from home'. If this is so, it is not surprising that a physiotherapist finds it hard to get the patient to open up about her daily life at home, let alone the intricacies of her marriage or family. Perhaps Ms Mahogany had better drift with the tide unless it is to be a question of a rather determined struggle.

Case 20 (Ms Mahogany and Ms Poplar) – follow-up

This is 'Georgeous Gussie' who used to attend three times a week at Ms Poplar's old hospital since the year dot. Somehow this patient assumes a different image although they both still agree that she is 'quite mad'. At Ms Mahogany's hospital she has recently had an osteotomy operation with quite a good result. This is amazing in view of the previous picture of a chronic patient addicted to a nonsensical supportive ritual and for whom nothing more could be done. She is now in a 'minimal care ward', a unit for patients who require a certain amount of skilled attention each day, during their convalescence, but who do not otherwise need to be in bed or to be looked after. In this setting, she is quite smartly turned out (a feat of nursing or her own achievement?) and is described as 'quite attractive'.

On the other hand she has written two letters. One is to the doctor at the previous hospital. The other letter is to Ms Poplar, addressed hilariously as 'Dear Sir or Madam'. Sir or Madam is asked to intervene in the present regime of treatment. Her dosage of Dopa, for post-encephalitic Parkinsonism, was cut down during the period of surgery and the Parkinsonian symptoms are worse. Would Sir or Madam tell the present hospital to restore her Dopa to the proper dose again.

Case 29 (Ms Sycamore)

This is another old man with an above-knee amputation – Mr Hoskins. He is 84. He was in two years ago for an osteotomy on his hip and did very well. Since then he has had a colostomy (why?) and a prostatectomy operation twice. The first attempt did not work properly. Now he has had an above-knee amputation for arterial disease and this is, once again, the problem of how long you keep trying. He is different from some other cases in that he can do his exercises very well, when he tries, but he is not inclined to make any effort now. He pretends not to know Ms Sycamore when he is in the mood, but she is confident that he is not genuinely confused at all. They all had a douche of cold water when he went to Roehampton for provision of an artificial limb. There, they thought that there was no realistic possibility at all of achieving this. Meanwhile, Ms Sycamore ploughs on and Mr Hoskins, when he wishes, achieves proud feats on the pulleys and parallel bars. Usually he will do nothing.

There was quite a long discussion about the role of the ward sister in this. This has a real day-to-day bearing on the case of course; it also served to illustrate, at a slight distance, some of the attitudes and problems of the physiotherapists themselves. Mr Hoskins is her pet. Sometimes this can mean that the patient is being infantilised for the gratification of some so-called 'mothering' predilection and there seems to be little doubt that Mr Hoskins would, in consequence, rather stay where he is than go anywhere else. This would be an important factor militating against learning to walk and moving off. This is reinforced by the gloomy reputation of the hospital to which he would be most liable to move, if he makes progress. Acknowledgement was also made of the intuition of a skilled and experienced ward sister in judging which patients are not going to last long and who should be left where they are, for that reason. It is significant that the case is presented, and talk of mobilising and moving Mr Hoskins has blown up now, while the ward sister is away on holiday.

We discussed this 'mothering' business. There is an obvious polarity between the function and impetus of the nurse and the physiotherapist. Whereas the nurse has a job of caring and looking after, nurturing and so forth, the physiotherapist always has her sights on activity, independence, and moving forward. The nurse's unchallenged dominion over the patient's bottom was noted in passing. While it is an important function of a good mother to help her child learn to walk and, ultimately, develop complete independence, there is much doubt and difficulty in recognising this at the emotional level. Members of the seminar were inclined to see many of their functions, in contrast to those of the nurse, as being the function of fathers, with an emphasis on striving and physical achievement as well as straight bossing about. So we come back to the previous laugh about 'Dear Sir or Madam'. The point here is that they experience much of their work as being at variance with their ideals of femininity. To put it differently, they discover, in their own deeper aspirations, the wish to keep their patients as babies, an aspiration which the nurse can easily satisfy but which is a particularly inappropriate interference with the work of the physiotherapist. They have to employ more mature ideas about mothering, ideas which are more of an amalgam with their preconceptions of fathering.

Eighteenth meeting — Wednesday, 27th September, 1972

Case 30 (Ms Mahogany)

A man with an ulnar nerve injury several months ago who was treated at Newcastle by surgery but has not had any physiotherapy. Later he had a neuroma removed and has had a little physiotherapy during the last month at Newcastle, until referral to Ms Mahogany's hospital now, as he has moved to London. There are several problems in this random case (the last one she saw this morning).

Firstly, some problem around organisation, responsibility and authority in the treatment, in that Ms Mahogany lies somewhere below the head physiotherapist who is an authority on hand injuries and devotes herself to them. She takes over and interferes the whole time and has directed Ms Mahogany to delegate the treatment of this case to a younger colleague, who should get the experience.

Secondly, there is the question of the head physiotherapist's suspicion that all these cases are self-inflicted.

Thirdly, why has he not had physiotherapy before, so that the whole thing is very badly neglected and with a very uncertain prognosis in consequence? Should this be investigated and by whom? Should Ms Mahogany speak to her colleague in Newcastle.

Fourthly, the prescribed treatment (prescribed by head physiotherapist) will involve several hours a day of daily attendance, for many months. The man protests that he will have to go on to half pay or worse (a civil servant) and so all this has to be evaluated.

A problem that emerges, cutting across all this, is the pattern whereby they never feel really entitled to question about matters personal or psychological but reckon only to be able to 'pick up' what information they can on the job. In this case the information is really necessary *before* getting onto the job, or even before being able to establish that the patient is going to attend for the job of treatment.

Ms Mahogany herself doubts the necessity or worth of such intensive treatment, as the case has now been so neglected and since it seems to be hard to arrange. She does however acknowledge the exceptional experience of her chief in this area.

Case 31 (Ms Elm)

During her work as liaison officer. This is just a matter of some thoughts about 'a rather pathetic, weedy little postman who fell over on his bottom' a few months ago and has had severe bachache and trouble ever since. He seems 'perfectly genuine' and 'backs are always difficult' and unpredictable. He responds reasonably well to treatment (uncertain, but probably heat and exercises) but relapses again when the treatment stops. Ms Elm was present when he was being seen by the surgical registrar. She reported the state of affairs and was very astonished that her report was received with the acid comment, 'Very convenient!' Normally this registrar is a very nice, kindly chap and Ms Elm is puzzled why he placed this interpretation, so hostile to the patient, upon her report. He was also rather unpleasant and crushing to the poor little patient. The situation is modified by the fact that he actually did prescribe a corset and some other line of management which seems reasonable and appropriate in the circumstances, so that Ms Elm did not feel that his actual management was now side-tracked. But she was puzzled and rather anxious about all this. The registrar is a nice chap and she could easily have tackled him if necessary.

Case 32 (Ms Oak)

Her last one this morning. A question of keeping her (the patient) back to finish her treatment and therefore returned to the ward a little late for lunch. This would not matter as there would be 28 other lunches to serve in the ward. The patient has already been kept in hospital several weeks longer than she (the patient) really wanted, on Ms Oak's request, in view of the necessity for more physiotherapy and the benefit to be gained from it. This is a case of rheumatoid arthritis and it is doing reasonably well, making good progress and Ms Oak has felt all this to be worthwhile. The incident is simply a study of something about Ms Oak keeping the patient, or keeping the patient back, for more treatment than she might otherwise have had, without her (Ms Oak's) particular sort of concern. Ms Oak again wonders about the quality of this excessive (?) concern of hers. We also note a repetition of the theme of two weeks ago, where people got strangely upset if their lunch was late.

Case 27 (Ms Oak) – follow-up

Ms Oak also makes a follow-up report on the case of two weeks ago. It has all blown over, The patient did stay a week longer, has now gone home and will return when the new out-patient/day unit is opened. The row with the sister is forgotten as quickly and as mysteriously as it developed.

Nineteenth meeting – Wednesday, 11th October, 1972

Case 33 (Ms Elm)

Ms Elm's case itself continues her work in the out-patient clinic, liaising with the surgical people. The woman patient entered with a weird gait which the registrar totally failed to notice. She drew his attention to it, whereupon he got her to walk so that they could examine the gait. It was 'the rolling gait of a hip' but he then got her to walk on her toes and on her heels, whereupon the gait became normal, so far as Ms Elm could see. The registrar proceeded to dictate a note to the secretary, describing the gait with reference to the weight being swiftly removed from one side or the other, I have forgotten which. He sent the patient home to have a month's rest in bed.

It had already been made clear that there was a big problem for the husband to have time off work if this woman had to go to bed or, indeed, come to hospital. He would have been there outside that day. She had also had substantial physiotherapy for her back to no avail. It is clear that Ms Elm thinks, with good reason, that the weird gait is proven to be hysterical, that there is something going on between husband and wife, and that some appropriate referral, or other management, should be initiated. After th patient left Ms Elm made some very feeble overtures around the point which the registrar seemed to overlook and so she dropped it – she is 'only the physiotherapist', after all.

After due wound-licking around this, I pointed the parallel between man-and-wife and physiotherapist-and-registrar. She sees clearly that this woman's peculiar gait and collapse, flat on her back, is really tough on the husband. It is harder for them to see that their own peculiar stance of, 'I'm only the physiotherapist', can be part of a secret war, in which nobody has more than a hollow victory, between physiotherapist and doctor. As I see it, Ms Elm first notices the gait, which the registrar missed. Thereupon *he* is able to *demonstrate* that it is hysterical but he then, for some peculiar perverse reason which I think is linked with the collusion between them, is determined to blind himself to this and to make a somewhat impotent gesture instead. He is a nice chap and they get on well together but nevertheless, beneath the surface, she holds him in contempt and he knows it. This is absolutely at variance with all the apparent situation about their status. It also brings out the almost inconceivable (to them) idea that the doctor might envy the physiotherapist (for her professional, personal and sexual attributes).

Case 34 (Ms Elm)

Another problem of a chronic patient, old Mrs Strauss who has moderate generalised osteoarthritis. Some time ago Ms Elm managed to get her to progress from elbow crutches and a great deal of fuss, on to sticks and less fuss. But when Ms Elm sent her back to the surgeon Mrs Strauss 'managed very cleverly' to fall over in the doorway and 'had to be caught' by the doctor. So they get her back. Ms Elm continues to see her around, treated by other people. She has just found out that she is getting some desultory treatment for one thing and another. She comes up by ambulance three times a week, which bothers Ms Elm a lot – and is then given a rather derisory treatment and left to get on with it herself. This contains all the usual problems about the chronic patient who is attending long after the time when any good is being done by the treatment. Ms Elm has verified from the social worker that 'everything possible is being done' for Mrs Strauss and indeed 'she has a lot going for her'. The problem is simply that she appears to be dependent or attached in some way to this treatment and Ms Elm feels that it is 'making a fool of physiotherapy'. This business of making a fool is what struck me as the central thing, continuing from the first case, where problems of status and derision between the professions involved are on our minds.

Why is it so difficult to tolerate the notion of a placebo treatment, and to allow students into the notion to gain experience of it? The problem is partly due to Mrs Strauss being a very unlikeable person.

Another important issue arises from Ms Elm's belief that this treatment is not doing any good, even as a placebo. The patient is not enjoying it and nobody enjoys having her. Ms Elm feels that the present arrangement may be preventing Ms Strauss from some more appropriate adjustment as well as being an inappropriate and annoying way of occupying physiotherapy time and space. If Ms Elm really does think this and if she is right, what can she do? Various forms of confrontation, amiable or belligerent, are possible between the physiotherapists and the doctors, who keep referring the patient back. Ms Elm thinks that even if matters were amicably settled, this woman would somehow get referred back a month or so later.

Twentieth meeting – Wednesday, 18th October, 1972

Case 11 (Ms Oak) – follow-up
On Anna. A couple of months ago she was chatting to Anna the day before the ward staff nurse was getting married. Anna astonished her by saying something like, 'You come with me and we will have a baby together'. There is some uncertainty about Anna's broken English and she may, on one version, have said, 'You, me, baby together'. At any event, Ms Oak rather panicked, pretended not to understand, and has tried to keep her distance since then. She still greets Anna and keeps in touch to make sure that her chair is comfortable and that the nurses know how to adjust it, but otherwise she has kept off.

Now Anna has raised fresh complaints about pain in her knee and has raised these complaints via the consultant on his rounds, so that Ms Oak is invoked to give some exercises. There would have been plenty of opportunity to raise this directly with Ms Oak if Anna had wished. Ms Oak has been doing quite a lot of work with a younger woman with acute rheumatoid arthritis in the next bed and Ms Oak suspects some jealousy.

She is very worried about the possibility of Anna's erotic excitement at being handled by her and wonders whether she ought to keep off the case or not. It is very hard to know how far Ms Oak is revealing her own panic, as against the possibility that she is judging, quite accurately, that this patient is inflammable. The notes reveal that 10 years ago, at Stoke Mandeville, she was diagnosed as having had hallucinations and she had caused quite a bit of trouble, with allegations of improper conduct towards her by a doctor. More recently, Ms Oak had reported in the seminar some minor near-delusory

133

state in which the patient got very excited about grievances of an imaginary kind.

Ms Oak has openly remained very impressed and interested at what she feels to be my interpretation, early on, about her taking the role of mother for this patient. What is now revealed is the complexity of this role as mother and how it rubs in the fact that women may have ideas of having babies together, without this necessarily being a barmy idea brought in by a psychoanalyst.

Case 35 (Ms Mahogany)

A woman of 57 with a Colles' fracture at the wrist. The plaster was removed two weeks ago and the usual routine of exercises commenced, daily at first but now three times a week. At the very outset, Ms Mahogany noticed a furtiveness about this patient when asked about her occupation. It turns out that she is on the Disablement Register and works only sporadically, as a clerk (?). She is supposed to be on the Register because of having had a neuroma removed from the ankle some years ago and it is baffling to know why she is supposed to be disabled. She walks perfectly normally.

She does her exercises badly and with difficulty, except when supervised, and makes heavy weather of it all. Incredibly, she has obtained a home help who does the housework and even does the shopping as well. Ms Mahogany finds herself caught up in the role of task-master so that all questions are directed, in a somewhat accusatory way, as to why the patient does not do this, that and the other. The problem is how to get out of that position and into a real investigating/diagnostic one. It takes us also to the recurrent question of whether the physiotherapist has a real licence or brief to take the patient into a private room and find out what the devil is going on, rather than simply having to slip in questions conversationally, in between the exercises. We await follow-up on this one.

Case 36 (Ms Oak)

A man in his 50s with symptoms of a cerebral tumour of very recent onset. He had a craniotomy performed only a few days after the onset of acute symptoms, so it has all moved very quickly. Before the operation, he was quite explicit that he would know afterwards whether it was 'vicious' or not. However, since the operation the usual conspiracy of silence has descended. He has made rapid progress towards 'recovery' with his exercises and they were hoping to bundle him off home while the going was good. He, however, refuses to go home until he is 100 per cent. They do not seem to be able to recognise this as a confrontation about the issue of prognosis.

Meanwhile, the wife has had a breakdown and went into a mental hospital on the other side of London for a day or two. Otherwise she sits at the foot of the bed weeping.

Again, we await a follow-up to see how this will develop. What line is Ms Oak going to take and with whom? Should she blow the gaffe to the patient or should she have this out with her medical colleagues?

Twenty-first meeting — Wednesday, 25th October, 1972

Case 13 — follow-up

Ms Poplar spoke about the situation at her hospital in its last days. Her Italian athlete is now the only in-patient left while the out-patient jobs are only trivia. She sees him as caught up in, and reflecting, the hopeless apathy. In particular, it is something about a state of mind which she describes as 'waiting for Mecca to come'. In this situation, with the whole staff of nurses etc and only one patient to look after, they had, during Ms Poplar's holiday, managed to let him develop a bedsore. His nails are 'as long as Dracula's' and nobody thinks of cutting them. He doesn't get washed . . .

Ms Poplar herself is attending various job interviews, usually offered the post but doesn't know what she wants yet.

Thence — discussion of what the physiotherapist ought to do when involved with a treatment which she does not believe in. A sense of lacking scientific methodology discussed. Ms Poplar and Ms Elm have both been prevented from doing an MSc by the poor status of physiotherapy as a basic training. Ruminations about how far this is linked with it being a woman's profession — men 'would run it differently' and 'be more scientific'. One member felt different since she was married — or rather insists that everybody else sees her differently, since she can call herself 'Mrs'.

Male physiotherapists are somewhat scorned as being either blind or queer but at the same time there seems to be a sense that they are more efficient and 'know what they are doing'. I made some interpretation that there was some pressure to look for and exploit an external difficulty, as between physiotherapists and doctors, or women versus men, as a defence against the doubtful character of physiotherapy itself. Like psychotherapy, it involved working rather on hunches, subject to impressions and hope, in an area of great uncertainty. However much scientific validation is desirable, the general character of the work will still remain the same and carry the same problem.

Another thing that came out of this was the aspiration to be able to 'do the whole thing' — diagnosis and planning of treatment (eg examining and assessing the extent of a chest condition) which seemed to me rather unrealistic, but it is hard to be sure. Certainly, there is great resentment of the cases referred by doctors with detailed instructions (often fatuously inappropriate) contrasting with the way a doctor referring to another specialist does not tell him what to do.

Twenty-second meeting — Wednesday, 1st November, 1972

Case 11 (Ms Oak) — follow-up
Again Anna. The main new point is that the pain in the knees has now disappeared without any particular treatment. Ms Oak takes this as confirmation of the suspicion that the symptom was psychologically generated — possibly by jealousy of the other new patient. There was some further discussion about whether Anna could 'really' have meant it when suggesting that they make a baby together — was it 'lesbian'; was it something that might really belong to a mother/daughter situation; do daughters have that sort of feeling about their mothers?

Ms Oak has been wondering whether she should have pursued any of this more directly with Anna. We are struck that she has herself become more awkward and self-conscious with the patient since there was the open discussion here of her role as mother to this woman. People are not always liberated by insight — sometimes it is the opposite.

135

Case 37 (Ms Sycamore)

A very new physiotherapy student had a meniscectomy some months ago in her home town but had little or no physiotherapy — probably because she developed German measles and glandular fever in the hospital. Ms Oak now has her for physiotherapy and finds that the disability is out of all proportion for a girl of 19, let alone a physiotherapy student. She has been noticed around the department as having a 'bizarre gait' and the Principal already has it in for her. The Principal is known to get it in for people, in a rather spiteful way, and last year, there were some unpleasant episodes where students were chucked out.

Ms Sycamore is able to joke with the girl about her slackness but is unable to take it further. She has also tried to chat to her on a friendly basis, but the girl is very unforthcoming. There was some question as to why she went into physiotherapy and, allegedly, it is something to do with her friends having gone into it six months previously.

The problem is partly that of being both teacher and therapist, having loyalties to the department and the profession as well as to the patient. This, as well as the usual traditions and habits, prevent her from any direct approach to this girl and her difficulties. All thoughts move towards reassurances about confidentiality and trust etc and away from any confrontation with the anxieties: (a) is the girl suitable — physically or psychologically — for the training that she is starting? (b) what, in reality and in fantasy, is wrong with the knee? Was a bit left behind, did they do the wrong one . . . ?

Case 35 (Ms Mahogany) — follow-up

The woman with the Colles' fracture who is on the Disablement Register. Ms Mahogany has enquired in the social work department and found that this woman is not on the Register yet but is trying to get on it. She obtained a home help, without any medical recommendation, simply by confronting the social workers with her arm in plaster and complaining a lot. She also complains that she falls over a great deal, allegedly because of her ankle disability, which no one else seems to believe in.

We get a fairly clear sense of this patient who is fully committed to getting on to the Disablement Register, but the seminar is bogged down in its anger with (a) the patients who pursue these perks, in contrast to all the poor old things who never get anything; (b) the doctors and social workers who collude in turning healthy people into invalids. Stuck with all these feelings, it is not difficult to see why Ms Mahogany cannot get very far with the case, which has indeed now stopped treatment and disappeared. Before she disappeared, Ms Mahogany — who actually seems to be very friendly and untormented by it all — had arranged occupational therapy for the woman in order to pursue these questions of what she can and cannot do. This had apparently gone very well. The woman had appeared to enjoy it and gave Ms Mahogany a jam tart she had made, at her tea one afternoon.

Another detail — her broken wrist did not occur from a fall due to the ankle but because the neighbours insist on feeding pigeons and there was shit on the stairs, on which she slipped. Much laughter.

Twenty-third meeting – Wednesday, 8th November, 1972

Case 36 (Ms Oak) – follow-up

More of a recapitulation than a follow-up since only Ms Mahogany was here when she discussed it before. This is the man with the cerebral tumour and the problems around telling or not telling him the terrible prognosis. We get a clear sense of the awkward situation and the particular interesting detail of his (a) inability to do upstairs, in the ward, what he could easily do down-stairs in the gym; (b) his announcement that he was not going home until 100 per cent cured. Meantime his wife has been in and out of mental hospital for a couple of days in an anxiety state . The present follow-up is to indicate that he did at last go home and we do not really know how they are managing. The social worker has been in touch but no services have been required. Ms Oak herself appeared to carry out a mixture of reassur-ance, jollying along (admiring his smart suit), on the one hand, and halting attempts to confront and ventilate his anxiety and disappointment, on the other hand.

We exposed something of the defensive hospital system, whereby the whole experience is fragmented amongst different people, moving from ward to ward etc, and the physiotherapist may be (or may feel) the only person providing continuity – although she can slide out of it too, if she wants to, very easily. We also discussed what might be encountered if you do not slide out of it – it is not a question of honesty simply being the best policy. If you are going to be honest with this man, you will have to face his anger and disappointment, as well as his sadness and anxiety. There may be something about physiotherapists being possibly the most obviously 'fit' people around the hospital and therefore all the more subject to envy by patients.

We discussed 'bloody-mindedness' and came to see that it had a literal significance here: and as well as the actual physically-caused mental disturb-ance, pain, confusion, headache etc, produced by a brain operation, there would also be the rest of the iceberg – the huge realm of fantasy about people poking about in your brain-box and feeling literally bloody-minded.

Behind all this is our sense of Ms Poplar's twin sister, whom we gather has a related condition. I have the feeling that the seminar will be working on one cylinder until we have all cried together over this – and this reflec-tion reminds me that I did also confront them with the sense that they may feel quite a lot of pain, bewilderment and anger from the defensive system used. While acknowledging the awfulness of what is to be faced and acknowledging the pressure on all people in hospitals to resort to these arrangements, they may have to come round to a sense of the inefficiency of these defences and even the extra pain that they cause. We note the enormously wasteful drop-out rate in nurses and physiotherapists, so we see that defences do not work all that well.

Case 38 (Ms Sycamore)

A boy of 18 with a knee; a compensation case (?). This is another thorough-ly fragmented case, where nobody knows the whole story and indeed, there is even some sense that important lumps of the notes are missing. She recalls his referral with the weird diagnosis of 'bruised infra-patellar fat pad', which the seminar found rather hilarious. The story is unknown but Ms Sycamore took over the treatment a few days ago in the absence of the student who was treating him – this student herself being one of a long line.

Last week the boy had an MUA (manipulation) or EUA (examination under anaesthetic). It is probably quite important that she did recall it only as an MUA for which nobody could see any possible rationale, whereas the notion of an EUA for diagnosis could well have made sense. In other words she saw him as having been subjected to something which made no sense to her. Everything she said about his management produced strong disapproval from somebody. He spent two years under treatment and quite a lot of time with a back-slab, which resulted in the disappearance of his quadriceps. Then they removed the back-slab and of course he fell all over the place.

Last week, after his EUA/MUA, the notes record him as having a 'maniac episode' — presumably some sort of post-operative confusion or delirium but there seemed to have been a number of stages to it, lasting into the next day. Anyway he had to be kept in for a day or two. The psychiatrist saw him and decided there was nothing wrong.

We get a sense of the utter fragmentation but with lively hints of thorough medical mis-management, guilt; and fear of being persecuted in some way by this patient ('? compensation case' — with litigious implications). Ought we to devote some thought to Ms Sycamore and her student? Can we leave it that she is just one more cog in the machine or is there something there that should be looked at more closely? In any case we await a follow-up now.

Twenty-fourth meeting — Wednesday, 15th November, 1972

Opening discussion led quickly to dying children and Ms Yew saying that it seemed to be easier to talk to them than to dying adults — that children seemed to accept their impending death much more openly and without fuss. She quoted children saying, 'Me next', when another child had died of a similar condition. Ms Elm agreed and connected it with some sense of feeling for family and for dependents when an adult was dying, as well as somehow indicating, to us, her sense of identification with the dying adult.

After some discussion of this I said that I heard Ms Elm indicating what was essentially what she in turn heard Ms Yew saying — namely that we find it easier to put up with children dying. At depth there is even an element of being glad the little beggars are dead. I linked this with the preceding discussion about students and youth today, and feelings about newcomers. This is not the whole story of our feeling about the death of children but it is today's emphasis — namely, that we feel somewhat as older children, hating the new arrivals and we can also feel as children bereft of their parents. We can identify with the devoted feelings of the parents, as a separate matter; but there is this very hard-to-swallow element of baby-hating — suddenly and startingly in sharp focus.

Case 39 (Ms Elm)
This involved the death of a young man, not actually her patient but involving her as a close colleague. This was a man of 22 who presented with an osteo-sarcoma following a football injury. He had an amputation a couple of years ago and it stuck in her mind that his mother would not (or, charitably, could not) have him home with an empty trouser leg. He had to be fitted up with a prosthesis, capable of exhibiting a shoe, before she could really bear him around. Ms Elm found this very alienating in the mother.

He died recently, having been married six weeks previously. A few weeks

138

after getting married he produced a lump in the chest. Ms Elm was in the staff commonroom when she heard him catch the colleague outside the open door and tell her, 'They tell me I've got three months . . . ', further calculating that this meant he would die soon after Christmas. She and the colleague both felt this dreadfully, although the seminar did not discuss much as to how and what the response actually was. He was admitted for a course of intravenous injections and actually died four days after the first one.

The colleague was full of concern for the poor young wife but the point of immediate interest to us is that Ms Elm felt much more concern for either the mother or the parents. She also spoke of wanting to write to them. After due discussion I voiced my sense that Ms Elm was expressing identification with the mother (a) in all the poignancy of a terrible loss, far surpassing that of the young wife; (b) but also recognising herself in the mother whom she sees as having some very nasty feelings about the son — wanting him only for narcissistic purposes, not really able to back her motherly concern with fulsome love. The point that came through to me was some sense that 'mother love' may be a thin affair, if the predominant feelings are those of an older sister.

Before this, Ms Elm had spoken again of her picture of the terrified mothers holding the children and afraid to let them walk, when the plaster is taken off their fractured tibias. I felt I was being spotted as an over-anxious parent who inflicts his anxieties on the children and this led me to bring this out, with reference to my interpretation about groups, right at the beginning today. Perhaps I was inflicting upon them my own anxious preoccupations about groups, rather than really helping them, in the appropriate way, with an anxiety that was relevant to the matter in hand.

Continuing Ms Elm's case — she then said that actually her concern was with the father, who seemed such a nice chap and had been very appropriately concerned, eg trying to get some sense out of the orthopaedic surgeon when the boy was going to get married. The orthopod had ensconced himself in some position of 'not disclosing anything without the approval of the patient' who had himself of course not been told the prognosis by this orthopod. It was evidently the radiotherapist who told him the truth, leading to the staff-room episode described below.

Case 40 (Ms Yew)

Ms Yew had raised similar feelings about children with polycystic disease and mentioned having reached this point with a 13-year-old lad who had himself said, 'I can't stand much more of this', a few days before he died. While acknowledging the kindly side of it (more, indeed, than they were claiming) I pointed out their sense of the link with the mother who cannot stand the boy with the empty trouser leg, the lungs full of cysts, or whatever it is. After all this had been talked around, there was some silence. I had previously taken up Ms Yew's remark about it being pointless to try to be chatty with this boy, who could hardly breathe.

I pointed out the possibility that somebody might nevertheless go there and just sit — not be chatty. Ah, but there are nurses . . . Ms Oak remarked on the way we are getting more silences in the seminar lately and wondered what it was about. I said I thought there must be times when the right thing to do was to shut up — and indeed I felt that there was not too much place for proliferating clever talk, in the context of what was being discussed.

Only after all this did we get round to some sense of more genuine mother love and the unimaginable poignancy that was involved in the death of one's child — and our need to sidestep this.

Case 41 (Ms Yew)
An instance of the over-protective mum. A girl of 14 with cerebral palsy has been in growing need of a tendon operation for the past two years. The mother has constantly resisted this — 'We don't want any of that, do we?' Eventually she and the girl were got before the surgeon who turned out, rather to everybody's surprise, to be very successful in managing and reassuring them, so the girl is going in for the operation soon. The mother insists on talking about it as a holiday. Ms Elm spots the selfishness and hostility of the mother, as well as some peculiar wistfulness about the whole ordeal, expressed in calling it a holiday. Ms Yew, on the other hand, does remind us that the mother really is terrified of something even if, of course, she is wishing her fears on the girl. It is a question of terror, not mere selfishness. It may be a terror that is also wished for. I saw this as connected with their wish/expectation for the surgeon to be knife-happy (Ms Mahogany's openly expressed fears).

The general wish to set up male surgeons in some such way emerges, as well as some pleasurable submission to their knife-like attentions. My reference to this as also involving the fact that the physiotherapists were women and the surgeon a man, was too much to take and perhaps anyway it did blur the central point at issue — namely the mixture of fear and wish that the surgeon should be a frightening butcher.

From this we also got on to the addiction to an organisation in which treatment is fragmented and distance is maintained. Nobody had demurred when Ms Yew described the set-up in her hospital as one in which all the staff treat all of each other's patients — ostensibly one big happy family, but sounding more like a chaotic situation in which nobody is really involved properly. I linked this with the same lack of astonishment at Ms Oak's initial announcement of her set-up, with daily rotation of staff. It turns out that they all 'realised' that Ms Yew 'didn't really mean it' and that 'there were good explanations', that people 'really did have patients of their own' etc; it had already emerged that Ms Oak's set-up involved changes that might be at intervals of a few months rather than a few days. But I pointed out that simply listening to what they say, rather than to what they are supposed to mean, we do get this picture of a frighteningly chaotic situation and a rather gay addiction to it. I connected this with the idea of the operation as the holiday and with Ms Yew's own contention that she would 'be quite happy to trot along' to the surgeon if necessary herself. I see this as going along with, rather than directly opposed to, Ms Mahogany's fear of the knife-happy surgeon.

Twenty-fifth meeting — Wednesday, 22nd November, 1972

Case 37 (Ms Sycamore) — follow-up
This is the physiotherapy student with the knee — following a cartilage removal at another hospital — before she came into physiotherapy a few weeks ago. She is making hardly any progress with the treatment and the Principal is hovering about, full of enmity. The problem of anxieties around confidentiality is very obvious — almost too obvious. Although

there may be problems of confidentiality about the girl's private affairs, there is a great deal of peculiar cloak and dagger behaviour around the immediate question of her treatment, her knee, her progress and her suitability for the profession. Although she has a peculiar gait which has attracted attention all around, they still pretend that her bad prognosis as a physiotherapy trainee is a matter of secrecy between the two of them and to be kept from the other senior staff. Actually, it is public knowledge, although the one person who may not really know is the girl herself; she would, of course, know unconsciously. It linked very much with the problem last week, of secrecy, confidentiality etc, about the prognosis of patients with grave illnesses.

Ms Teak and Ms Yew — perhaps speaking as new people — pressed for the need to clarify the actual condition in the knee and the possible need for the opinion of an orthopaedic surgeon. I queried whether this was some sense of the need for a man around. In any case it is not clear whether this ambiguity about the diagnosis is preserved as a further way of side-stepping the psychological problems: on the other hand there is some sense that it may be a flight from the psychological problems to orthopaedic surgeon in the hope that he will bale us out. It is clear that unless some sort of confidence and ability to talk is established there will be some other pickle, whatever the result of an examination under anaesthetic, or whatever.

Case 42 (Ms Poplar)

This is the problem in her new job and not a particular patient. She has started this new job in a large gynaecological department where she is head physiotherapist with just one assistant. This assistant qualified in physiotherapy before Ms Poplar was born. Ms Poplar says she is a very nice person, a swinger, very gay and with-it, but there is an impossible gulf between them regarding the nature of the work. This woman has carried out a routine for decades, involving a great deal of trivial physiotherapy. In particular it seems to be a question of 'pre-ops and post-ops' — for operations where the anaesthetic is only five or 10 minutes, eg for a D & C. Similarly, there are ward drill classes to prevent thrombosis in the legs, although all the patients involved are up and about the day after their operations and have in fact to be sent back to bed to do their exercises! This routine fills the colleague's time. Ms Poplar is faced with the double problem of being new and not wanting to rush like a bull at a gate, changing everything and upsetting everybody. The nurses all expect this routine and collaborate with it. Moreover, if she does do this Ms Poplar seems to think there will be just about nothing to do and has already had to take a detective story to read to kill time. In contrast to her previous hospital where she 'had to do everything', the staff here are excellent in all branches and morale is high.

The underlying problem which will really determine the outcome is the psychological disturbance around and about all this gynaecological illness and surgery. Not only is there a constant sequence of suction terminations of pregnancy (which appear to be simple and quick) but there are also extremely unpleasant saline terminations of later pregnancies which upset everybody and which Ms Poplar certainly finds very unpleasant. It also comes through that, in her own bald-headed way, she has already shown awareness, and responded to her awareness, of some of these problems. She has tried to talk to people about the nature of their operations instead of blindly doing pre-op rituals. She also mimicked annihilatingly the Oxford-accented houseman who seemed blithely unaware of the problems of a Chinese patient having a saline abortion.

So we shall have to wait and see, I think. The seminar members were inclined to devote themselves to the staffing problem, ie the problem of staff deployment and the sense that Ms Poplar could easily talk herself out of a job, there being really only work for one person. Another version was that this was an ideal place for Ms Poplar and one student and thence a discussion of whether this was not really a suitable job to plonk a student into.

Case 36 (Ms Oak) – follow-up

This is to say that her man with the cerebral tumour has died. They had a very nice letter from the wife to say that he had died peacefully at home last weekend, thanking everybody for their efforts etc. We do not know any further about the unresolved questions as to what he was told about his diagnosis and prognosis.

Case 38 (Ms Sycamore) – follow-up

Another knee – this time the man with the (?) compensation/litigation problems. This is the emphasis presented, although nothing was ever very convincing about it. He is the young man who was being trained in hotel work (hotel management?) and who had a 'maniac episode' one weekend immediately after an MUA (manipulation under anaesthetic).

The essence of the follow-up is that Ms Sycamore had been able to get absolutely nowhere with his exercises during the few days she was treating him. She is chagrined to find that different students both before and after her period, have been able to do very much better. Things are still far from well but considerable progress has been made and the chap is, at the moment, away for a week at home with his family in Somerset. There are two main theories: (a) that he responds better to a younger physiotherapist, and, more particularly, to somebody he perceives as a beginner, needing his help – in the same way that the most junior nurse on the ward can sometimes get on better with a difficult patient than her more experienced seniors can. There was some laughter at the notion of Ms Sycamore as 'an older woman'; (b) Ms Sycamore was conscious of being much more gentle, kindly etc than the students, who were brisk or even brusque – certainly much more firm and emphatic in their expectation that he should get on with it and move his knee.

Again, we get the question as to whether the diagnosis cannot be taken further but this time Ms Sycamore is emphatic that he had a full range of movement during the MUA and the disability is mainly psychological. This certainly applies to the non-effort that goes into the exercises she tries to get him to do.

For me there emerged two questions: firstly, the question of diagnosis. How does the physiotherapist pursue her evaluation of either of the above theories or any other theory she has about it? Secondly, can we not look more closely into this business of what goes on between Ms Sycamore and this patient? She has told us explicitly about her own trick of being sweet and gentle in order to get the men under her control. There is a clear sense of this chap rendered impotent by her kindliness, which was recognisably reflected, moreover, in a certain 'kindness' of the seminar towards Ms Sycamore. In effect, this kindness leaves her in the position of being gently approved of here and, ultimately, rendered quite ineffective. There appears to be some polarity, especially in today's material, between Ms

142

Poplar and Ms Sycamore, representing the belligerent as against the sweetly seductive approaches. Ms Poplar was surprised and incredulous, as she sees herself in more agreement with Ms Sycamore than anybody else.

There was a final emphasis on compensation neurosis, miraculous recoveries when the money is paid etc. Ms Teak wanted to push this and 'produced a case' — really an old anecdote from some remote experience of this sort. Somebody else mentioned the case of the 'crippled patient' who had been 'followed by a private eye' with a cine-camera, revealing him to walk normally when not watched. We have to distinguish this rare sort of malingering from other variations. In the main, I am becoming known as a firm disbeliever in this syndrome. I have gone on record as not believing it!

Twenty-sixth meeting — Wednesday, 29th November, 1972

Case 43 (Ms Oak)
When on weekend duty she was giving physiotherapy to a post-operative cholecystectomy, who was producing copious purulent sputum. Something made her speak unusually sharply or feelingly about the evils of smoking, whereupon the patient, a middle-aged woman, challenged Ms Oak as to whether she recognised her. Ms Oak did not, but the woman recognised her. Ms Oak had treated her little boy four years ago. The child died — I am not clear whether it was in the period of Ms Oak's care or not. Anyway, this woman had four children with spina bifida and they all died. So, in effect, this woman told Ms Oak that she had something to smoke about. Quite a catharsis followed, with some weeping and Ms Oak herself was quite moved. She feels that the episode was beneficial, on balance, and the patient appeared more cheerful, more mobile etc when she saw her again later in the week. But what interests Ms Oak appears to be the nature of the impulse that made her speak in the way she did. She is inclined to see it as 'putting my foot in it'.

She describes how she tends to avoid seeing (ie avoid noticing) the parents who are standing there behind any child she is treating. She remembers a child quite vividly but has no recollection of the mother. We are left wondering how far (Ms Lime's emphasis) this woman recognised in Ms Oak somebody who could be approached. On the other hand we wonder how far it was Ms Oak's own initiative, either because she recognised a patient in distress or whether (my suggestion — incredible to the others) Ms Oak, at depth, really recognised this woman for the person she is. We are all preoccupied with dying children and how the mothers feel about it at the moment. Ms Oak may have been dredging up something that she dimly did recognise. There was some other discussion about aversion from smoking as a silly or filthy habit etc but this was rather in the service of maintaining that Ms Oak's remark was something which could have happened with anybody at any time.

Case 44 (Ms Elm)
Brought with some diffidence, after quite a bit of hesitation on everybody else's part. The diffidence is because it is a private patient, with a tangle of feelings about that. A nice elderly woman aged 75, in a very expensive flat off Bond Street, 'needs mobilising'. The referral is quite 'correct' via a neurologist and via a private physiotherapy practice Ms Elm works for sometimes. Although liking the old lady, Ms Elm is also confronted by a

couple of ghastly over-dressed daughters and, returning from abroad some weeks later, a son. Ms Elm examines the patient and finds symptoms of Parkinsonism. She gets her head bitten off by the GP when she mentions this on the telephone – he denies this diagnosis. Moreover, in the family there is a great denial and opposition to it, although the son is delighted with Ms Elm's diplomatic formula that she 'presents features of Parkinsonism', to which the son adds, 'But she doesn't actually have it'. Considerable progress is made at first and Ms Elm and the old lady are delighted. Reversals promptly occur as upsets develop with 'the children' (grown-up children). The son is busy manipulating his mother's drugs, putting her on and taking her off and we wonder where on earth the doctor is.

The first and main thing that strikes us is the terror of death and disease in these people but also our sense that Ms Elm may be too ready to hail the marvels of treatment and too slow to be 'with them' in their fears. She tells us that she herself has a family who appear to live for ever (an aunt of 95 being mentioned from this last weekend). But we are really at the beginning of the problems of how to see, more precisely, *what* are the fears of death: there appears to be some emphasis on shame and dirtiness, linked with something about helplessness. There is a family commotion when mother is unable to get up to answer the door.

There is also a commotion about some hired help, in the shape of a woman called Mildred. Mother hates the idea of having this woman in and Ms Elm sides with her. Ms Sycamore, amongst others, sees Ms Elm as being a bit too hostile to the daughter and unwilling to recognise the real need and possible benefit of having Mildred around.

Right at the end, we get a much clearer sense of the way Ms Elm is caught up in sibling rivalries and the triumph of being able to help mother *while the others cannot*, ie militating towards their continuing to be unable to help her.

This sprang from Ms Lime's suggestion of a possible way of working by involving the family actively in the treatment, rather than as undesirable spectators. By contrast Ms Elm on her last visit had found herself having to lie on the floor to demonstrate exercises for the son to teach Mildred, before she herself could escape from the flat. We now see that if she could have got the son or daughter on to the floor, *without unpleasant feelings of triumph and contempt*, it would have been a possibly more constructive device.

We also touch on feelings about money, fantasies of being bought. We eventually learn the son asks Ms Elm if she can give him help with his back! An implication of all this is that if physiotherapists are really to push for the benefits of domiciliary work, they must sharpen up their diagnostic skills and their techniques of intervention in the family scene. Which one of all these people in the household is the best one to tackle?

Twenty-seventh meeting – Wednesday, 6th December, 1972

Case 37 (Ms Sycamore) – follow-up

On Janet, the student with the knee. Two simultaneous developments. Firstly, Ms Sycamore had some talk with her about her suitability, etc. Secondly, the Principal has dropped her from the school. Ms Sycamore tried to tackle Janet about her suitability and her general desire to continue the course. She found herself up against cotton-wool – vague uncertainty

144

and indecisiveness, ready to agree to anything, or, at any rate, to conceal any disagreements. She asked her why she had gone into physiotherapy and the reply implies that her school put her in for it by default, as being one of the very few 'respectable' jobs for a girl from a nice school if she does not go to university or teacher's training. However, this was instantaneously mixed up with Ms Sycamore's implications about her own school and her own choice of career. From some sense that, 'It was just the same with me . . . ' I rather uneasily felt that there were one or two genuinely relevant details and a whole string of assumptions, with a failure to differentiate herself clearly from the girl. However, Ms Sycamore did compare and contrast the girl with her own sister of the same age and was struck by Janet's extreme immaturity.

Meanwhile, the Principal appears to have decided, understandably enough, that Janet must go. The explanation given is that she is evidently not motivated to do physiotherapy or she would otherwise have been better motivated to do her own exercises for her own knee. Ms Sycamore does also record that she herself failed O levels, which was her way of resisting the school's plans for her and Janet might be doing the same thing with her knee. Could Ms Sycamore have put such an observation to Janet?

The seminar are ready to settle into a fight session against the Principal. However, they had all agreed, when I asked, that they saw no hope at all of this girl succeeding in the profession, ie they agree with the Principal. Ms Teak reminded us that senior teachers in universities etc all seem nowadays to welcome the notion of the older student, the one who has gone away and knocked about while making up his or her mind. It is doubtful whether we can altogether blame the Principal for the failure to deal with this girl with a little bit more imagination. Ms Lime would like her to have been sent for some counselling. In the absence of a counselling service there is some discussion of whether the social worker could have been used — remembering that this is a patient, as well as being a student. I put in a plea for some attempt to recognise from amongst the colleagues around the place, which ones are good with particular sorts of problems. Perhaps the social worker might be and ought to be better at talking to people than the orthopaedic surgeon; but it is important to recognise which colleagues are good at that sort of thing rather than relying on what they are supposed to do. Behind the question of the suitability/acceptability of this student I thought there was also the question of how far they can accept and use the discordant aspects of themselves — for example, in this instance Ms Sycamore's own indecisiveness.

Case 45 (Ms Mahogany)
This is a hot case because she had just taken it over, although it is actually three years old. A man of about 50 with sudden severe rheumatoid arthritis a few years ago, very severely disabled. The problem presents as one of getting him out of the department and off treatment, which is not progressing. The context is that he gets his wife to do everything for him, manipulates the staff and sets them against each other. In recent months, the wife has been presenting with pains in her neck and back too, increasingly severe, and she also has quite serious heart disease although it is somehow played down in the discussion. All these problems are made worse by his weight — about 16 stone. He is a big chap but this does represent extra obesity.

It appears to centre around the fact that he has been attending twice weekly for about three years to swim in the physiotherapy pool. He enjoys

145

swimming about and it is his only real experience of mobility and activity, but he does not push himself and is basically unco-operative in any attempts to use the pool for physiotherapy techniques. They cannot seem to get anywhere with him and have been trying 'to sack him'. When, at last, they got the rheumatologist to make some such decision recently he promptly snapped an extensor tendon in the hand and had to be admitted for repair of this. Now it is a last-ditch stand with the senior registrar determined to have him out, various other wards refusing to take him in and Ms Mahogany wondering what is happening. She appears to be quite tranquil about it, repeatedly emphasising that, to her surprise, he is a nice chap when you talk to him but she does wonder . . .

The seminar take against him in a big way, seeing him as fat, lazy, exploiting and manipulating. They are full of sympathy for his poor wife who has turned into a sort of hand-maiden, bathing him, taking him to the lavatory and attending to his every need although he is perfectly capable of doing most of these things for himself. Moreover, Ms Mahogany finds herself pushing him along in his chair and working the brake for him, similarly doing every little thing that he could perfectly well do himself. The point, moreover, is that it is a dereliction of physiotherapy to be doing all this for him: the whole idea is that he should be learning to do more for himself rather than less and less. He is very well-off, well-equipped so far as mechanical devices, gadgets, etc are concerned but there is resistance to getting extra help in the house or using the district nurse because he prefers his wife to do all these things for him.

As the wife is now cracking up it may be the wrong moment for the hospital to abandon his treatment. Actually, the plan is to have a six weeks gap to review the effect of this, ie to demonstrate whether there is any effect of his attending the pool. The seminar are more than usually critical of this man whom they see as greedy, lazy and exploiting. They find it hard to look at the collusion all around to keep him as a fat baby, like a pudding. I also had the recurrent feeling that this is another version of the way the doctor-men are kept silly and ineffectual by the colluding women (physiotherapists and nurses) who *appear* to be submitting and being left with all the work. Somehow the doctors are not enabled to get on their feet and be effective on the job and are very much the silly babies that Mummy has to give way to.

There are untouched questions about prognosis and fear, in both the man and wife. What about her heart disease? Is it really a question of reading him homilies about being inconsiderate? And what about what it does to you to be struck down in your prime by painful crippling disease? Is there any place for physiotherapists and nurses to have a real role as 'being kicked about', to give him some expression for his wish to retain power and authority? If they duck out at this moment is this really going to help the wife who will have to carry it all?

I did finally feel that the turning away from prognosis and anxiety were the most important areas for the seminar and we did not really get into this properly. Another detail: he has a grandchild with spina bifida, who has had to have both feet amputated. (Can this be true?)

Twenty-eighth meeting — Wednesday, 13th December, 1972

Case 46 (Ms Teak)

A tall gym teacher aged 42 has had at least two operations on each knee for removal of patella and medial meniscus on both sides — at another hospital which has closed down. Now presents with *backache* and clearly wants an operation on her back and will be satisfied with nothing else. She is admitted for investigation. Is being seen by a neurologist and psychiatrist and no further orthopaedic opinion is sought, because the diagnosis is that 'the problem is not physical'. The psychiatrist has one hopeful interview but, after his second, decides that he can do nothing at all with this woman who 'refused to admit to any problems psychological'.

The patient is sent down for physiotherapy to the knees, one of which is swollen. Ms Teak can't do anything right. She sent the porter up with the chair to bring Miss M down and was ticked off as she could walk. Miss M derided Ms Teak as being only able to do what she is told. Ms Teak 'treats the knee' and it is only with some difficulty that I can interest the seminar in what this treatment is. It turns out to be a mixture of exercises and ice packs. Anyway, this is not at all what is wanted and the patient has now left hospital, very dissatisfied with everybody. Ms Teak feels extremely uncomfortable about the situation, with a feeling of failure, which is different from more straightforward surgical failures.

At first the seminar are bemused by the notion of acting in the image of the psychiatrist and want to know what psychological enquiries Ms Teak could have pursued or tried to. She did indeed ask a variety of questions and got nowhere. With difficulty, the seminar are brought to attend to their own type of access to the patient. Then it is realised that here is a woman who wants her back attended to and is not going to be satisfied with some substitute treatment to the knees. It is noted, with some interest, that Ms Teak did not think of examining the back whereas others felt they would have been too curious to resist this temptation, if nothing else. Then there is the question of her wanting an operation and her ability to turn everything round into maltreatment. Do we need to recognise that the wish is for maltreatment of some sort? Is it possible for the physiotherapist actually to dispense some acceptable form of maltreatment? Alternatively, it may be possible to diagnose that the person wants to be hurt, mutilated or whatever and then to have a clear sense that *this* is one's reason for opting out of the situation - if one does not wish to fit in. Actually, there did seem to me to be room for at least thinking about treatments that would be some-what unpleasant rather than going for the treatments which are pain-relieving and soothing, like ice packs.

And what is the particular significance of the patient as gym teacher? Is it too close to physiotherapy for comfort on either side? And why was Ms Teak deflected from looking at the back?

Case 45 (Ms Mahogany) — follow-up

Mr S has now been discharged from hospital and banished from the pool. It is again elaborated how all the staff seem to crumple in his presence and it is puzzling to know quite what this process is — crumbling, melting, shrink-ing? There is now some sense that the staff turn into babies; there is an inability to be responsible. This seems to reflect last week's picture of this patient as commanding everybody with his babyish dependence. Even the discharge is rigged. He is taken on a home visit but the person escorting him is told not to bring him back! Somehow this was achieved and he was left at home. Afterwards, everybody is anxious lest he fall over there and the hospital be liable for damages, having dumped him in this way.

Although Ms Mahogany does confess to annoyance with him at times, for his duplicity and playing people off, she is nevertheless very friendly about him. On the other hand, Ms Elm and Ms Poplar are infuriated by the picture of this man getting women to do his dirty work and wipe his bottom. It is only with difficulty that they come to realise that it is specifically that sort of thing that upsets them. We gradually get a sense of emphasis and pattern to these details: of how his lavatory has to be just the right height for him to sit on while he shaves himself; his refusal to have elastic which will enable him to pull up his own pyjama trousers. He has been induced to let the district nurse come and bath him, instead of his wife, although everybody thinks he could really manage himself anyway.

We did at least make a step forward in exposing particular specific feelings about lavatories and different parts of the body, as distinct from some general sterilised medical image of all-parts-of-the-body-being-the-same in the eyes of the physiotherapist, striving to achieve function.

Case 44 (Ms Elm) – follow-up
She is still seeing her old lady and trying to confront her with feelings about getting old – hitherto a taboo subject.

Case 47 (Ms Poplar)
Just five minutes at the end. She is giving 'foot and ankle exercises' to a 'repeated abortionist' – a woman with habitual abortion who is now in for bed-rest through her pregnancy, for months on end. Ms Popular has some minimal contact with the patient's husband, who is in the same line of business as Mr Poplar. The patient chats compulsively to Ms Poplar about her husband's absences on business, which legitimately does take both husbands abroad a lot – but Ms Poplar often goes too. The chatting is amiable and optimistic.

Now Ms Poplar has just been given an awkward confidence by the house-surgeon, at a unit party, when he told Ms Poplar that the patient's husband left her at the beginning of the year and is suing for divorce. What is she to do with this unmentionable information? Is it even true? The houseman is a funny chap who seems to believe the patient is in love with him. (A further complication: Ms Poplar had not even noticed that this brings in problems about the parentage of the pregnancy which is being so carefully preserved. Apparently the husband did want a termination at the beginning.)

We had to leave this in the air but I did note it as having a bearing on remarks earlier in the afternoon. Ms Lime had been advocating an 'attitude' in which a climate is maintained, in which confidences can occur, and in which it is possible for the patients to declare their psychological problems. This would contrast with a situation in which the physiotherapist has to start turning on a psychological enquiry, which is out of keeping with her normal activity. Ms Poplar is always at the ready and admits quite frankly that she is impelled all the time by curiosity and therefore tends to drop hints and openings amongst 'innocent' chatter. Now we have an example of some of the difficulty this atmosphere can get you into, whereby you pick up confidences and information in a way which is informal and does not lend itself to any professional management very easily.

148

Case 48 (Ms Lime)

Really presented only in initial conversation. A 10-months-old spastic baby.
She has not treated one before and was looking for advice from Ms Yew
(from paediatric unit). The mother is only about 20 and has another three-
year-old who is very active, a bright boy who runs around the department and
gets into everything. Usually this child is left with grandma. It emerges that
baby and mother live with the grandmother and are separated from the
father. However, there is talk of father getting a place and them all going to
live together again. The mother is understandably timid about the handling
of this spastic baby, seeing him as more fragile than he really is. A lot of the
work is, of course, done through and with the mother and it is a question of
working on her, rather than the baby. Behind this we get the question of
involving the grandmother and thence — on my instigation — the father.
The seminar are tempted to get lost in helpless feelings about not having a
psychiatric history, not knowing the whole story of the separation etc. I
point out the possible indication for getting grandmother and/or father into
the consultation as part of the basic physiotherapy programme. Might it
not be possible to arrive at diagnostic impressions from actually seeing his
engagement or grandmother's engagement in the clinical work, instead of
having to take it the other way round — getting a history and then wondering
whether we can involve him. Might the father be better than the mother at
mobilising this child, but, if he isn't, something important will be that much
clearer.

Case 44 (Ms Elm) — follow-up

On her elderly private patient. This has now turned very sour. Whereas
she was formerly a sweet old lady with unpleasant daughters, she has now
turned into a nasty old woman, querulous, demanding, spiteful and grudging.
Ms Elm has decided to space the visits out to a week apart, instead of twice
a week, on the grounds that the old girl was becoming more dependent and
there was no future in this. This produces an emergency phone call early on
Sunday morning to Ms Elm's flat, although Ms Elm was actually away. So
an extra visit was put in on Monday and she is going in again after the seminar.
Then she is away for Christmas for a week or so. Ms Elm had been trying to
get the patient to understand more of her feelings about ageing and death,
which was obviously a sore point. She is not prepared for the tangle of
emotions aroused. As a physiotherapist she also suffers feelings of wounded
vanity and helplessness as there is the prospect of labouring through all this
— in parallel with the patient's own feelings about ageing, slowing and the
need to work out how to get out of her chair, in stages, by numbers. It
suddenly comes through, in flashes, that Ms Elm was caught up with the
idea of cure, new hope etc, and has not really had the idea of having to sit
this through while the patient gets worse and eventually dies. All this also
fixes us with the renewed question of making people lose their sure-footedness, with only an uncertain possibility of being able to take them through
to something better afterwards. This links further with the reluctance of
people to bring forward cases at that point — nobody wants to turn 'an
ordinary case' into a problem.

A further detail coming to mind about Ms Elm's case — around being
grudged a cup of tea by Mrs B, but coming early today and being given
one by the paid companion. Tête-à-tête in the kitchen the companion

declares how horrible it is and that she is leaving and how Mrs B expressly forbade her ever to offer Ms Elm a cup of tea. Does this link with another free association about the way Ms Elm was once given sherry by the son who, while saying he would not have anything himself, actually kept going to the cupboard and taking secret swigs of whisky, in secret from his mother? Is Ms Elm therefore being regarded like the plumber, a menial; or is she regarded like the son — there being some link between mother's grudging of a drink to both?

Case 49 (Ms Yew)

'Not really a problem' (but see the end!). A three-year-old girl who has had an astrocytoma removed from the thoracic spine. The tumour was not operable but she has been treated with radiotherapy and appears pretty well. Following a recent fall she gave up walking and is now slowly getting going again. The view seems to be that this is not a physical disability and she is attending for physiotherapy. She is brought by both parents whom Ms Yew keeps describing as 'super parents'. She has attended three times. She shouted all the time during the first visit, less during the second and much less during the third and is now getting 'quite good'. What does a 'super parent' or a 'good child' mean? Is it something to do with being the sort of patient or parent who does not trouble the physiotherapist with awkward questions or shouting? Ms Yew is vague about the prognosis. When confronted, she seems to agree that it is very bad but nothing is very open. The seminar are particularly concerned about whether the present symptoms may actually represent growth of the tumour. Conversely, if this really is a psychological commotion, where exactly is the disturbance? The seminar finds it very hard to swallow the notion of a child of three being capable of hypochondriacal anxiety although Ms Yew, more experienced in this than the others, agrees readily. She also laughs that many of these little children know exactly how to play their parents off against each other. She sees this child as not wanting to resume walking (for whatever reason) and her tactic is to get her moving by any means possible. She will certainly walk if she is pushing a trolly but quickly declares that she is 'feeling poorly' and wants to sit down. There is also some question of her being constipated — but again, the seminar can only see that this might be a parental anxiety. They cannot see that a child might have anxieties about it herself.

Going across all this is an appalling family history. These parents have already lost two other children from totally unconnected causes. One died from gastroenteritis, another died of spina bifida and now there is this tumour. All this came out in a 15-minute discussion and shows what trouble you bring on yourself once you start asking.

Thirtieth meeting — Wednesday, 10th January, 1973

Case 48 (Ms Lime) — follow-up

This is the 10-month-old spastic baby with a three-year-old brother and the mother. In the background are grandmother and an absent father. We had wondered about bringing in these other adults. The mother now says that she has decided to leave the husband. Actually they were not living together anyway. There is something about him always being unreliable and, in particular, never having been able to have anything to do with the spastic baby. Ms Lime emphasises her impression that there is still a good deal of love felt. It is not a bitter or nasty separation, on the face of it.

The theme also continues around Ms Lime's need for advice, information and support in her work with the child. She has never treated a spastic baby before and there is a lot of practical know-how, tricks to learn, as well as facts and information, eg about standards to be expected at different ages and so on. This was carried over towards the notion that she might attend the mother's next consultation with the paediatrician. This is in the same hospital group but in a different building a mile or two away. For someone in her department, this would be an unusual step although, of course, not intrinsically an unusual thing for a physiotherapist to do, within her own hospital.

For me, this question of what sort of partnership could go on between Ms Lime and the doctor, and the larger question of what sort of help she can glean and need, linked with the question of what might be salvaged of the marriage and the question of what this mother needs in the way of support from the husband and other people. She evidently has quite a lot of professional support from the welfare departments and the remaining problem really is that of the husband. I still wondered whether the physiotherapy treatment was the one area in which the husband might appropriately be brought in. Would it be a help to him and to the child in future to build up some basis of contact? If we do have a sense that the marriage may have foundered on the birth of the spastic child, is there some basis for hoping for a sort of 'marital treatment' based on accommodating the father to his damaged child. Incidentally, the child was said to have been damaged in birth trauma by asphyxia, or anoxia.

Case 50 (Ms Mahogany)

A large forbidding university reader (in her 50s) who has a ruptured Achilles tendon. It has been repaired, she was discharged from hospital a week or two ago and this is now about the out-patient physiotherapy. Ms Mahogany found her a cold fish. She responds in a flat, daunting way to any attempts at humour and is closed to any other form of conversation. She 'walks atrociously', makes hardly any perceptible progress or effort towards her treatment. Ms Mahogany feels up against it and finally exploded when she saw the woman walking around the department 'in a very bad way' that she had been specifically instructed not to do. To her surprise, the woman flared up, told Ms Mahogany she was a bad teacher and caused a nasty scene in public. Ms Mahogany is frankly afraid of the woman, also sorry for her and recognised that she (the patient) was at the end of her tether. On that occasion she had flopped into a chair unable to take any more. Ms Mahogany had been able to return to the situation and restore some sort of friendly semblance of co-operation but, basically, the impasse remains. She had sent the patient back to the physical medicine doctor (a woman) who had 'had too many psychos' that morning and 'proved feeble'. Thus the woman came back, with an additional request now for treatment of osteo-arthritic knees! During a few conversations Ms Mahogany had asked the woman whether she had much work and things to do at home. The woman had replied darkly that there were plenty 'of things'. Otherwise she had recounted some story of having 'always had trouble with the other knee' (on the good leg). She says that there is gout in her family and she knows she has gout although, when thoroughly tested last year at the hospital, gout was disproved. Ms Mahogany feels baffled at this 'unintelligent' sort of attitude in a sophisticated person. The seminar were not sure how far there was some sense of gout as being an upper-class disease[1] in image and this woman as being a superior, would-be special sort of person. Last year she was also supposed to have told the doctor that she thought she had a psychosomatic disorder of the knee and this sounds like a frank confession of psychological difficulties but we are not sure. We can't decide whether she is flaunting her depression and really does want to talk; or is a superior, arrogant teacher of teachers who finds it crushing to be a patient/pupil.

There was quite a long discussion eventually about the department ruling which forced her into shorts for treatment. There was a feeling that while it may be 'impossible to treat' this sort of condition in slacks, perhaps in retrospect slacks plus co-operation would be a better recipe for progress than shorts and the present state of affairs. It sounds as if Ms Mahogany was very nice about it and protected the woman's modesty with a dressing gown, cubicle to change in etc, but the feeling still comes across that there is some sort of degrading process going on in this treatment situation. So we are left with a number of different lines that Ms Mahogany might want to take up — the woman's depression, the 'things' at home, her arrogance and the painfulness of being plunged into a baby position learning to walk. Also general styles of management that might reduce the collision between the lecturer and the physiotherapist. I did raise the question whether there are patients who will not be suitable for physiotherapy and can be recognised. It was emphasised that, in this case, there is quite a lot of anxiety about the degree of disablement that might result if this[2] is neglected through apathy.

Case 44 (Ms Elm) – follow-up

Her elderly private patient. She is getting in a terrible pickle with this family. It is partly a tangle owing to feelings about fees, private work etc but even more, the problem of working in unorthodox ways, on the edge of the spectrum of normal physiotherapy. It is interesting to contrast this with the treatment of children where the use of games is absolutely normal. It is similarly 'all right' to use the opportunity of giving the old lady a bath in order to teach her the techniques of getting in and out of the bath and so on. However, this has slid into the role of physiotherapist as nursemaid and dogsbody. Ms Elm is never allowed to get away at a normal time, there is always some problem about her being allegedly too late or too early and the edges (or even the middle) of the session are invaded by different members of the family. In particular, the son is very pressing in his demands for Ms Elm to take him on as a patient and the mother jokes that he appears to have a crush on her. There is now another doctor in the picture and we don't quite know which one is the proper one. An arrangement for a joint consultation with Mrs B, Ms Elm and the doctor was aborted by Mrs B, to the fury of the son, who had come home especially from work hoping to see Ms Elm. The seminar have to take quite a strong hand in trying to strengthen Ms Elm into patterns of proper professional behaviour and to remind her of quite simple ways of behaving that could keep the situation clear. In addition to this, there is some question that perhaps she should withdraw from the case and certainly, that she should withdraw from all these tangles with the rest of the family.

There is a crucial paradox between her delusion of being indispensable to an old lady who is now 'dependent on her' and the actual reality of Ms Elm being shoved around like the most menial servant who is allowed no independence at all herself. We did not clarify or discuss any sense that the pressure to control Ms Elm and make her dependent is directly understandable as a reaction to the family's need for her, a direct attempt at reversal.

Notes
1 It isn't, of course, but the seminar were familiar with the popular myth.
2 In other words, there is real danger of serious physical disability permanently ensuing if this treatment cannot, somehow, be promoted successfully.

Thirty-first meeting – Wednesday, 17th January, 1973

Case 48 (Ms Lime) – follow-up
Just briefly to mention that her patient now reports the beginning of court proceedings for separation or divorce. The court ordered some reconciliation attempts but the husband did not turn up at the first appointment. This was a brief report of an encounter in a busy clinic.

Case 51 (Ms Sycamore)
An old man of 81 with a fractured shoulder a year or so ago (?) who 'did much better than the average run'. Nevertheless, Ms Sycamore dislikes him heartily and was very chagrined when the patient reappeared on her list just recently. It passes somewhat unnoticed that this differs from the more usual syndrome of disliking the patients who do badly. It only later becomes outlined why Ms Sycamore dislikes him so much and even then, it is not really clear. He has always been a very independent-seeming person and proud of it, full of good works and Christian postures. It is this latter element that alienates Ms Sycamore, who can't stand the pious complacency.

Now, with the reappearance, things are different. Over the telephone Ms Sycamore noticed that this man sounded desperate. In the treatment session, there was a lot of moaning and groaning, although she found the limitation and disability to be relatively minor, on examination. Incidentally, the case was first given to one of the students, as usual, but the student very rapidly had to ask Ms Sycamore about it and she thought she had better take it over. Ms Sycamore found herself drawing the man out instead of following the usual habit of jollying along. By this time the patient had dissolved into tears and quite a lot became revealed of his loneliness. He has hitherto propped himself up (a bachelor) by making himself feel needed and valued, whereas now, in old age and some disability, this device is falling apart. Ms Sycamore wonders what to do next. She does not really think there is any case for physiotherapy but fears that if she reports this back to the fracture clinic, the man will not be treated with kindly consideration. At present the plan is simply to go on with treatment. The patient has been referred back to the social worker whom he has known for 15 years.

In contrast to the familiar pattern of disliking a patient who does badly, this is an instance of disliking the patient who did well – 'better than the average run'. This may be connected with annoyance about this patient who, in other ways, sets himself up as better than the average run. Secondly, we have to face the bi-polar love-hate relationship with these disliked patients – that is to say, those of them that are kept on.

Then we get on to the recurrent question of 'popping in and out'[1] and other indications that, at first sight, suggest unwillingness to do the job properly. We got a feeling that Ms Sycamore doesn't really want to get down to it with this man. However, the opposite possibility emerges –

namely that the devices of physiotherapists, eg the habit of popping in and out and the ready-made arrangements for breaking off or keeping things shallow — all these safety valves do enable the physiotherapist to get in deeper if she wishes. She knows she has a way out. We can contrast this with Ms Elm and her private patient where she is in difficulty because she has been separated from many of her usual safety arrangements in an out-patient clinic. I was struck by the balance between the two cases: in one (Ms Elm) the anti-semitism; in the second (Ms Sycamore) the antipathy to one species of 'Christianity'.

Cases 52 and 53 (Ms Teak)
Some remarks about a couple of patients, a man and a woman. Following identical operations, the man whom she disliked beforehand and thought would do badly, has in fact done very well. Vice versa with the woman she liked, who has done badly. Ms Teak finds, to her amused surprise, that she now cannot stand this woman, who is such a pain in the neck with her treatment, whereas she feels quite pleasantly towards the man.

Case 54 (Ms Yew)
This emerges as one she was urged to report by her boss and Ms Yew herself is only very marginally involved. The problem is around a two-year-old quadriplegic — a case of neo-natal meningitis. She is quite an attractive-looking child, which does give a twist to the situation, but she is a complete vegetable, unable even to sit up, and will never learn even to talk. The problem presented is that the mother half wants her home but believes that she will murder her (by smothering) if she does. She has tried before but could not quite carry it through. The mother and the hospital staff fully believe that this danger is a great likelihood. The child is brought from a residential home by a nurse, and the mother sometimes/usually attends for the physiotherapy treatment.

The mother is a simple-minded young Welsh woman, unmarried and it is uncertain who the fathers of her various children are. The father of this one is Jamaican (?) but anyway, not in the picture. Her first child was removed into care, for unknown reasons, and she brings with her one baby of 10 months.

The seminar struggled to find voice for the feeling that this was a hopeless case and anyway, not an appropriate one to bring to us. This is not Ms Yew's clinical problem and our intention is not to discuss other people's cases sent up for discussion in this way. However, Ms Yew voices the thought that once you find yourself involved in these hopeless or impossible problems 'you have to try and do your best'.

My impression was that the best we can do is to offer some model of how to say 'no' and some model of refuting the unreality that you must always, supposedly, struggle on in the face of something impossible. The point here is that this woman has the equivalent of a still-birth on her hands and she is being conned into struggling with an almost imaginary problem of how she will want to murder the child if she has her home. All sorts of possibilities for analysing and interpreting guilt etc spring to mind, but this is a simple person and the one thing that gets across to her from the present clinical situation is that 'you've got to struggle on'. Trundling this child out to hospital for physiotherapy is not in any way helping this woman to detach herself from the 'still-birth' nor to face what has happened. There is a misconceived idea here of 'working through' and avoiding denial — some vain idea of helping the mother to distance herself while also involving herself in what is happening. Actually, the physiotherapists are providing therapy for the doctors and social workers who are unable to cope with their own problem. Physiotherapy is an absolutely false and misplaced notion in this case which is pushing the woman into the presenting symptom — the idea that one day she will be able to have the child home and will then want to murder it.

Interestingly, Ms Teak was actually courageous enough to voice the idea that this woman should murder the child. Horrifying and shocking as this thought is, she feels that it has not been at all clarified just why this might not be the best thing to happen. In other words, she is giving voice to the unconscious wish which she recognises in her professional colleagues — the actual wish that this woman is really pushed into doing what they want her to do. This is a crucial recognition, in view of the supposed efforts going towards achieving the opposite.

Around this, there are other somewhat unresolved discussions, about what people report to their colleagues about these seminars. Ms Teak and Ms Yew, for example, are always questioned and give some sort of report the next day, however brief. The others wonder if they are falling down on the job of propaganda. This led me to remark that in these discussions (as well as in referrals to physiotherapy) we may have to recognise at least two polarities: (a) the polarity of idealisation and the expectation of omnipotence — perhaps the physiotherapist or the Tavistock can solve impossible problems; (b) the polarity of wishing to lumber the recipient with something that is crushingly impossible — the wish to bring our seminar down as low as possible under a load of crushing problems. Again, of course, the physiotherapist must watch out for similar referrals to her department.

Note
1 This was an important session for us. It clarified a great deal about the way physiotherapists can curb proximity and intimacy with patients, by a technique of doing several things at once and creating reasons for popping in and out of cubicles. This usually causes irritation and mounting anxiety but can, occasionally, act as a useful safety valve that enables better work to be done.

Thirty-second meeting — Wednesday, 24th January, 1973

Case 51 (Ms Sycamore) — follow-up
Raising the question of why she feels enormously better about the patient she reported last week. She found herself able to be either amused or interested, rather than angry, with this man whom she still finds as unattractive as she ever did. Ms Sycamore's recollection of last week's discussion is of some general themes about love/hate; she seems to have gone away with some deliberate notion of 'looking on the love side'. This of course sounds desperately fishy and sidesteps some of the uncomfortable thoughts last week about why the patient might be unlikeable. What did come out is the sense that Ms Sycamore felt able to experiment with not popping in and out in the usual way. She was quite interested to find that she was able to avoid this. This led to further discussions about the terrific pressure to get out for cups of coffee if one feels imprisoned in a department. If one is moving

around from ward to ward there does not seem to be the same difficulty about doing three hours at a stretch. I had a sense that Ms Sycamore felt more able to be closeted with the patient, once we had been over and clarified her need to be able to get out, if she wants to. There was no actual need to keep popping out to prove it. Another point was to feel less imprisoned by supposed attitudes, within the seminar and around and about. The supposed attitudes would be the expectation that you should have only nice feelings about your patients, certainly not feel chauvinistic, superior, anti-semitic, anti-Christian, scornful etc. Even if we allow for ordinary human likes and dislikes, there is less sense that we might really sanction attitudes which could not gain any public approval. This, having been exposed, may have left Ms Sycamore feeling less imprisoned in 'having to have the right attitudes'. On the other hand, this theory is not supported by her own impression of herself as 'going back to look more on the love side'. Meanwhile, the patient has seen the doctor and the social worker and the plan is to stop her treatment in a week or so. Ms Sycamore will probably continue it on her own initiative.

Cases 55 and 56 (Ms Teak)
She went on to discuss another pair of patients. These are a pair of young women who had both had operations on their backs. Ms Teak also mentions her impression that all patients with operations on their backs get depressed afterwards.

The first patient, Mary, a nurse, has had a laminectomy and spinal fusion, which was done in something of an emergency, owing to rapidly progressing neurological signs. Yesterday, only a few days before the patient is due to be discharged home, Ms Teak discovers in conversation that home is in Penzance, involving a five-hour rail journey. The girl is very worried about it and, indeed, it seems most unsuitable that she make such a journey alone. This gets into other problems about her friends and family, from whence Ms Teak discovers that the girl, a nurse, had an illegitimate baby four years ago which had to be adopted. The family appeared to be very much in evidence, very much babying her with presents, which Ms Teak had previously thought somehow to be incongruous. The parents seem fairly accepting but a younger sister is apparently very unpleasant about the disgrace she has brought upon them all. This led to practical questions of whom Ms Teak should tell. She had no conflict at all about telling the ward sister but seems to be in a great dither about whether to tell the doctor too, or the social worker. Meanwhile, there is the problem of whether the girl should go to a convalescent home locally, rather than make the long journey home, where she may actually be very unhappy. Whom should Ms Teak tell and what should she tell? Also, what should she tell the girl? For example, the girl is given precise instructions how to take a bath or a shower and what positions she must not adopt. What about love-making? What about future pregnancy? None of these get a mention.

There was something about the girl not knowing she was pregnant until five and a half months and her parents not believing that she didn't know ('It happened at a party when she was drunk.') This pattern of not knowing, massive denial, infects the whole medical management. Suddenly, it struck me that there was crazy blankness about the conspiracy not to know that the girl had this history. How many doctors must have examined her and suppressed notice of the post partum changes that would be obvious?

Case 57 (Ms Oak)

We made the mistake of trying to hear this in the last quarter of an hour. She rambled circumstantially through the account and had to be stopped in the middle, after five minutes overtime. It centred around the mobilisation of a woman patient, following an operation, with a large hysterical component. It is a picture they recognise well — the patient who puts more effort and skill into being unable to put one foot ahead of the other than could be encompassed by an acrobat.

Thirty-third meeting — Wednesday, 31st January, 1973

Case 48 (Ms Lime) — follow-up

It now emerges that the missing husband has, since Christmas, been involved in robbery with violence and a hit-and-run road accident. He is now under arrest and will probably go to prison for a long time. Ostensibly the wife, the spastic baby's mother, sees this as promising to assist her divorce which her own mother had probably always wanted. However, Ms Lime has always emphasised that this woman herself appears to be fond of the man too.

Ms Lime had not gone with her to the consultation with the paediatrician. There was further discussion about the parallel problems of this woman's isolation and Ms Lime's professional isolation. Also some question of how this happens and what is the connection with the spastic child patient. This one patient seems to be preventing any of Ms Lime's other patients reaching the ears of the seminar. This is only partly because Ms Lime followed what she took (mistakenly) as the pattern here — namely that people tend to follow one case along.

Cases 55 and 56 (Ms Teak) — follow-ups

Continued from last week: the two young women with back operations. Following last week's report Mary, the nurse, became cheerful and resilient the next day whereas the other one, Joan, dissolved into tears and helplessness. To prepare for travel, they all went over to the hospital to collect Mary's things. Everyone there made a fuss of Mary. Then they got a taxi back and it poured with rain and Joan dissolved into tears. In the taxi she said she could not face the traffic. Although she is going to get married, she feels a painful contrast between her inexperience and Mary's apparent poise, savoir-faire etc. There was quite a discussion about the processes of sympathy, empathy, projection etc, including an outburst from Ms Poplar about the way women get together in 'hysteria', all ovulating at the same time etc. I thought this tended to obscure the specific see-saw aspects of it and the use of one person as the victim or repository of another person's difficulty. The behaviour of the nurse (equals physiotherapist, equals doctor etc) gets herself back into a superior position by projection, repression, denial, and simply by forgetting her troubles. We saw last week that Mary had a tremendous capacity for splitting, forgetting hysterical dissociation etc.

This whole discussion had been ushered in by Ms Teak frankly confessing the attraction of being able to get rid of in-patients, all the time. With out-patient work you are stuck with them till they get better, more or less, whereas the in-patients are always coming and going. She was raising, in a rather flippant if challenging way, the pleasures and advantages of that sort

157

of superficial work. I tried to take it up in terms of clarifying what are the strengths and opportunities of the position, in which the physiotherapist feels securely that she is not trapped. This links with the question of the advantages of being able to pop in and out, so that the physiotherapist does not feel claustrophobia. The hope of the seminar would be that people are able, by coming out here on a Wednesday afternoon, to 'pop back in again' more deeply, with mobility, not just getting lost. Is there a sense that Ms Teak did do certain things and perhaps could have done more — by virtue of the special short-term relationship with Mary? Behind this, there were two clear notions, linked together: firstly the feelings, linked with Mary's feelings about her baby given into adoption, of regret at the loss of each patient who leaves hospital, like an adopted child, or like a baby given away; secondly, the recurrent theme of hostility to babies, especially to sick ones — the sense of being glad to get rid of them which, at times, has emerged as the idea of even murdering them. Ms Teak herself had been quite frank in raising the issue a few weeks ago: would it not be better for the mother to murder her paralysed spastic child?

Somehow, all this led on to the themes of classes, group work and some specific problems about pelvic floor exercises and quadriceps drill. There was a clear sense, and hints of known evidence, that some people being taught quadriceps exercises do better if this is done in classes. In spite of the time-saving appeal and the possible benefit of competition as a stimulus to some patients, other patients do better if treated individually. This links, and is contrasted, with the question of pelvic floor exercises, following prolapse repairs, childbirth etc. Some of this is done in classes (especially in connection with ante-natal training) but there are tricky problems of intimacy and demonstration. Is it possible to demonstrate, or somehow really know, whether the patient is doing a pelvic floor exercise properly? Some of this had come from a belated recollection by Ms Teak that there had been a very telling episode with Joan. Before the operation and before being contaminated by any of Mary's anxieties (ie before Mary was admitted to hospital) Joan had been given a preparatory enema and escorted to the lavatory by sister, whereupon she had got into quite a panic and declared that her hands were paralysed. The physiotherapists were very intrigued, although not surprised by this reaction. Ms Lime emphasised that her approach is to assume that *any* procedure is going to be experienced as frightening or painful and has therefore to be explained in advance at some length. She is prepared to use an entire first consultation on preparation and explanation, without actually 'doing any treatment'. Other physiotherapists thought that patients would be angry and disappointed if they came up and went away 'without any treatment' and it is always necessary to send the patient away 'with something'. I was struck by the steady, if slow and muted, emergence of a sense that quadriceps drill might be experienced, in the mind, as no different from pelvic floor exercises and similarly, various 'ordinary' physiotherapy procedures might be experienced as startling and paralysing as a badly given enema. We are now slowly getting to the very charged question of what is felt about bodily contact, the laying on of hands, exposure and intrusion in private parts of the body.

Thirty-fourth meeting – Wednesday, 7th February, 1973

Case 57 (Ms Oak)
This is a woman of 39 with, I think, six children, who is divorced or separated. The physiotherapy has been following a laminectomy. This appears to have been 'genuine' – a disc with neurological symptoms which have receded after the operation. The problem was a terrible commotion when the physiotherapists attempted to get this woman walking again. After the neuro-surgeon had done his ward round and given the word, they made a start the next day. Pandemonium developed, with shouts and screams and hysterical dancing of feet, sitting on the floor and all the rest of it. It is clear that this woman has first-class neurological co-ordination and all the antics would have caused more pain than they could possibly have been avoiding. So it was simply a question of management and handling.

Ms Oak found herself in a pitched battle with this woman. Owing to another emergency she had to take over from the physiotherapist whom she was hitherto assisting (although actually a senior) and this was followed by accusations, from the woman, that Ms Oak had dismissed the first physiotherapist and was now treating the patient cruelly. There is no question that anybody believed any of this and all the staff were heartily fed up with this woman. The feeling was that the psychiatrist should be asked to come and see her but the neuro-surgeon obstinately refused to agree to this. He insisted that the first thing to do was to get her walking and all the rest of her troubles could be sorted out later. I am inclined to see this as not unreasonable and the hopes of what the psychiatrist might achieve strike me as thin. Ms Oak was obviously flushed, excited and distressed, gulping and searching for words. She was explicit that she was showing here the sort of strong feelings and belligerent challenge that she thinks was very much concealed behind the usual patter on the job.

On the one hand, this seems to be connected with the recurrent flair-up of anti-doctor feelings. It struck me later, with Ms Sycamore's case, that there must be a regular fury of the patient against the doctor who mutilated and operated – and this is projected onto the physiotherapist who is inflamed into rage with the doctor too. I also wondered if Ms Oak was somehow getting lessons in how to stand up *from* this woman. At the end of it she went to the neuro-surgeon and, although addressing him as, 'Sir', she did state firmly that she could not treat this patient. It does raise the question why this could not have been done in a more casual way. Getting her to walk was, in the event, not a matter of any particular physiotherapy skill. Maybe it could have been much more easily and happily done by the nurses, who know the woman, and the houseman on the ward, instead of invoking a new stranger called 'physiotherapist', as if only she can teach this patient to get out of bed. After a few days, however, it was achieved; the woman was walking normally.

Case 50 (Ms Mahogany) – follow-up
Ms Mahogany and the patient discovered that their husbands were vaguely in a related line of country. After the ructions reported last time relations appear to have become much better between them. Ms Mahogany is really raising the question whether this is somehow related to the row they had or whether it is related to something else, viz that Ms Mahogany referred the patient firstly to the orthopaedic registrar who was fatuous and vacuous (making facetious remarks about 'all you married women') and then referred

the patient to her GP. Ms Mahogany had perceived, quite early on, that the GP was very good and he certainly seems to have succeeded. He gave the woman butazolidine. He also confirmed the woman's belief that she has gout which she seems to want to believe although, in the hospital, they hold that this is a load of nonsense. Whether by prescribing the drug, or by diagnosing gout, or however he did it, he seems to have been successful. At any rate the woman made good progress with the walking and was discharged yesterday.

Case 58 (Ms Sycamore)

This is a woman with recurrent cellulitis (and septicaemia) of the leg. After the woman had nearly died on a number of occasions, the surgeons were forced to amputate below the knee. Since then, there has been terrible difficulty in getting extension of the stump. The quads are very atrophic whereas the hamstrings work well and the knee stays in flexion. The physiotherapists were given the job of straightening the knee out and this put them in a terrible position with the patient upon whom they had to inflict awful pain. They were then instructed to fit serial plasters. They did this to the best of their ability and Ms Sycamore is absolutely enraged at the critical, unappreciative attitude of the doctors. They keep looking over her shoulder to see what she has been doing and imply amazement that she has not got better results. In the event, they do not appear to have been able to get anything better themselves, when they have stepped in.

They then arranged an EUA or MUA,[1] which they had been reluctant to do because the woman reacts badly to anaesthetics. However, under EUA the knee had a full range of movement.[2] Eventually it did get moving, I think. This was the case that made me realise (in relation to the previous case) that the physiotherapist must have to carry a great deal of projected resentment of the surgeon. Ms Teak had already mentioned her suspicion that all patients are depressed after back operations but this case led, in my mind, to the recognition that all patients must be angry after all operations — in some measure or the other. Certainly after an amputation.

Notes
1 Examination or manipulation under general anaesthetic.
2 Implying that the deformity was due to muscle spasm (which could be caused physically or psychologically) and not to a bony lesion.

Thirty-fifth meeting — Wednesday, 14th February, 1973

Case 59 (Ms Poplar)

This was an episode that morning, in which she had made something of a snap decision to refer a case to the social worker. She offered this for criticism, in the context of the above discussion. A Trinidad 'girl', who turns out to be a woman of 30 with a daughter of 16 (?), ie she had her baby when she was 14. The baby was fostered with a relation in Trinidad and she has never been able to be pregnant since. She has been an in-patient, having pelvic short-wave, I think, for God knows what. Now, towards the end of the course, she evidently recognised Ms Poplar as someone you could talk to and told her that her problems are 'really in myself'. She then described her depression etc. This came out more or less as Ms Poplar and/or the patient were going out of the door and Ms Poplar was about to rush off to something else. She did offer the patient the specific possibility of talking to her about it again on Friday but urged the alternative possibility of going to see a 'very nice lady', the social worker. We think the patient did accept this possibility and we do not feel too bad about it, in the sense that Ms Poplar has her own door kept open too. But should she have referred at all at this point?

After some talk, in terms of whether you 'should or shouldn't' and a general groping for the 'right thing to do', I tried to focus the discussion on the specific features of the case. I refrained from mentioning at this point that the matter was suffused with feelings about giving away your children into adoption. I also clarified that the referral was about Ms Poplar's picture of herself as the social worker. The sense that this patient needed 'a very nice lady', whom we rightly guess to be someone Ms Poplar sees as more motherly — all this is something the seminar wishes to step around. An important issue arose here when I asked Ms Poplar whether the social worker was old, young, motherly, or what. The joke answer is that she is probably in her early or mid-40s which Ms Poplar obviously sees as quite old but hastily and jokingly altered to being 'in her prime'. This joins up I think with the final case (see below).

Case 56 (Ms Oak) — follow-up
The chief point is that the woman rapidly returned to normal walking and has gone back to work. We go over the rather blurred question of quite how she was got back on her feet. It appears partly to have been Ms Oak's determined confrontation in the parallel bars. But later that afternoon, the woman seems to have resumed walking in the ward — partly to go to the lavatory but partly to avoid having to go down again to see that awful foreign woman! There is something about foreigners in all this: Ms Poplar wondered if the woman was Italian (like her Italian man) but she is, in fact, Welsh. Again, we are so caught up with the pros and cons of whether you should or should not get emotionally involved that it is difficult to pull back a little and examine the nature of this emotional involvement. Is this a case of a woman who delights in driving a wedge between other people? Is it some specific problem between the disciplines and professions? Is the friction between physiotherapist and neuro-surgeon a symptom of the woman and her case or is it the cause of the trouble? Everybody seems to have been much more anxious than they have admitted about the urgency of getting this woman on her feet. It might have been more sensible to let matters ride for a day or two, instead of having all this commotion on the one hand, or thoughts of sending for the psychiatrist on the other. In the event, we hear that the neuro-surgeon made a special evening visit to come in and see this woman. Why, if he was so sure that there was nothing wrong? Ms Poplar underlines her shrewd sense that he was much more worried than he admitted or, maybe, realised.

Case 60 (Ms Poplar)
This hangs over from a few weeks ago and was hotter then. She is 'giving foot and ankle exercises' to a woman with a pulmonary valvotomy and a threatened abortion. The bleeding subsides very quickly indeed but then the husband comes in and 'has his dose' in the ward, weeping etc, believing the wife will die over this pregnancy. She is approaching 40 and there is no cardiac indication for termination. By this time both woman and husband are clamouring for abortion.

161

Ms Poplar has 'established rapport' already and decides to have a further talk with her. She learns that this woman has one child of 18 and no others, but has been very busy fostering other children all these years. Ms Poplar reads this as being the expression of a great wish to have another baby and proceeds to tell the woman that she herself had an open heart operation and had her own baby 'an indecently short time afterwards' — within a year I think she said. She thinks the pregnancy itself shows the wish to become pregnant. The patient had been 'on the coil' but then given it up because of some trouble and the husband was waiting for a vasectomy.

After this, Ms Poplar felt that she had intruded in an unwarranted way with advice and persuasion which she had no right to give. Certainly, we get a sense that she has been breaking all the rules and homilies. There might have been a clear case for providing the reassuring information that, 'I personally have had a heart operation and had a baby afterwards. If you really want the baby you can see from me that it's all right'. However, it is obvious that she got carried away far beyond this.

The real twist of the knife is that the woman was not pregnant at all and that these were menopausal symptoms, for which she had been receiving hormones. These hormones had given rise to a false positive pregnancy test. So now Ms Poplar not only feels that she broke all the rules but that she 'looks a proper Charlie'.

We now have to face the question of what this woman was up to and what were the anxieties that turned Ms Poplar on. Again, the seminar grope about for general rules pro-con giving advice. To me the issue really is what suddenly made Ms Poplar break all her own rules. I think — and this is what links it with the first case — and the combination of the two cases did lead me to speak out — that this is all something to do with very strong feelings about other people's babies. Again, we have the same theme of fostering. There is not only the question of wanting babies but there are also questions of violently not wanting them. There is all this talk of abortion. The husband certainly did not want her to be pregnant. Ms Poplar did spell out some suspicion that perhaps these people really do not fancy the idea of being in their mid-60s before a new baby would grow up and be off their hands. Within all this, I thought that there were particular issues that somehow stirred Ms Poplar, and stirred the patient, about the menopause. There is something very grim about the joke earlier on. When is the prime of life? Is it death to be 40 or does life begin then when you get rid of the children? Afterwards it struck me once again that behind all this there is all the ghastly ambivalence about the death of children.

Thirty-sixth meeting — Wednesday, 28th February, 1973

Case 61 (Ms Oak)

Another case of a man with an inoperable cerebral tumour, whom she has been seeing since last week. We are mainly dominated by the perennial question of whether he knows the prognosis, what has he been told, etc. She is trying to teach or improve his walking, for which he requires a tripod. However, he noticed a walking stick hanging at the bottom of the stairs near the department and has become obsessed with the idea of being able to use it. Ms Oak is clear that he is simply not able to do so and certainly would not be safe to be left with a stick alone — he would fall. His balance is bad, apart from the actual hemiplegia. She promises to try and get him on to the stick but she feels that with the very bad prognosis, there is no point in making enormous efforts to achieve this end. We are preoccupied with the usual discussion about what the doctor has decided to tell the patient, what is the physiotherapist's place in the scheme of things, how much initiative she may take, etc. We also get a clear sense of hiding behind this and there is quite a strong suppression of enquiry in the seminar too. Nobody asks whether the man has had a craniotomy or X-ray therapy or what. There may be very obvious signals as to prognosis, diagnosis, etc but we do not really want to know that much about the situation.

There is also the question of specific anxieties about dying – and about living on. What is the social/family situation? What about the particular point at issue – the man who says, 'I am not a child you know'. There are problems here about the humiliation of being taught to walk, future humiliation and anxieties about passivity, dependence, infantilisation etc. Many of these anxieties have not so very much to do with the fear of dying and need some much more specific recognition. They could apply to a case of some non-lethal illness equally.

After this work is done, people are able to develop some practical thoughts.[1] Ms Elm points out the desirability of teaching this man mat-work, and exercises towards control and co-ordination – looking ahead to the time when he is unable to walk and will need to move about in bed, and so forth.

Case 62 (Ms Beech)
Brought forward with inexplicable[2] reluctance during the remaining half hour. Lady in her 60s with a facial palsy. The physical medicine specialist has prescribed that she attend daily for electrical stimulation and exercises. Her first visit was with her daughter-in-law and some friction appears to have developed because Ms Beech excluded the daughter-in-law from the tiny cubicle. The treatment lasted 20 minutes, instead of the 30 minutes the woman had expected, and this was also questioned and resented. Subsequently, relations improved and she learnt a bit more about this woman. She has a daughter who has had a hysterectomy, followed by depression, leading to admission into mental hospital. There is now some problem of confrontation between mother and daughter – the mother has been unwilling to face the daughter in her (the mother's) present condition but now the daughter has been coming out of hospital and visiting the mother. Ms Beech is struck that it is a question of poor mother, not poor daughter. The woman quotes the doctor as having told her that she will definitely get better and there is a daily inquisition as to whether any progress has been noted. Ms Beech does not see any but is somehow driven to pretend. She had this case on her mind when she was discussing Ms Oak's case – the problem of getting into this atmosphere of pretending that things are getting better when they are not. This case has only been going three weeks and could of course get better, but nobody knows.

Ms Beech has made unsuccessful attempts to see the doctor, who appears to be totally inaccessible. She does not even know what he looks like and he is carefully surrounded by secretaries, nurses, receptionists, etc. Ms Oak makes it clear that she would knock on his door and see him, without messing about, if she wanted to. Ms Beech had asked her superintendent about it – the superintendent obviously feels caught between the two and sounds weak and ineffectual. There is quite an atmosphere of everybody sparing everybody else – Ms Beech did not want to push the superintendent too hard. This seemed to me to have its reflection in the patient and her family – all these women who do not quite know how much they are leaning on each other. Ms Beech mentions that she is about to be moved off to some separate part of the hospital where she will work in total isolation. She seems to welcome this herself — vaguely, smilingly linking it with some sense of herself as trouble-maker. Ms Oak warns that this might be unpleasantly isolated — she herself (Ms Beech) appears to look forward to it. What do you do when a patient quotes somebody, whom you cannot get to see, as having said something that you think is nonsense? They all think the whole treatment is nonsense anyway, but this doctor is said to be somebody who likes his prescriptions to be carried out without question.

The session actually began with some mention of the appearance of behavioural sciences on the new curriculum for the training of physiotherapists. This is a big step forward even if it is only in name. There was some further discussion as to what had been/might be written about such seminars as these.

Notes
1 Careful attention to primitive anxieties then allows the emergence of the professional competence, which had been temporarily submerged.
2 Inexplicable then — but quite easy to understand a month later.

Thirty-seventh meeting — Wednesday, 7th March, 1973

Case 63 (Ms Poplar)
The point of the case is that the woman gets her angry and confused. The patient is described as 'a typical middle-aged layabout' who has recently had some gynae operation (salpingectomy) and is having physiotherapy for sacro-iliac strain — heat and exercises. This is making very little progress and the patient keeps deluging Ms Poplar with details of her sexual antics. She has been married several times and keeps regaling Ms Poplar with the endless gory and bizarre details of her sexual goings-on, with hermaphrodites, admirals and heaven knows what else. Ms Poplar feels, each time, that she cannot stem the flow which continues as she gets out of the door and she wants to scream at her, tell her not to be so silly, to act her age, etc. The woman lives in a hostel for wayward women and has been thrown out of it because she lit a fire in the wastepaper basket. She was thrown out of somewhere else for some other sexual antics.

The seminar do sense that behind Ms Poplar's dislike of the woman there is some sort of affinity, whether it is on the basis of 'there but for the grace of God' or whatever. Ms Poplar does recognise something of herself in the patient who has this pattern of running full tilt into a brick wall. Otherwise, in thinking 'there but for the grace of God' she adds, 'Yes, but it would only be in about 30 years' time'. Since the woman is 42 this would imply Ms Poplar at the age of 12 and the seminar blandly ignore this until I point it out in another context. What struck me was the continuity between this case and Ms Poplar's last case, where we got the same theme of middle-age. Clearly there is some problem of bizarre fantasies and anxieties about middle-age as some horrible sort of decay, with change or deterioration of the innards, linked with ideas of bi-sexuality and some unspecified ideas (this I did not voice) about compulsive sexual strivings which are supposed to put it right. (Last time it was a question of getting a baby; this time it appears to be a question of getting a penis.)

The difficulty is to establish some line of connection or division between

164

the sort of insights and speculations we have about this situation on the one hand and the actual clinical job on the other. I feel this problem is connected with the way Ms Poplar is pushed into producing sensational anecdotes by the absence of cases from everybody else. Somehow it did lead on to a discussion of the undercurrents that may go on in more ordinary cases of quadriceps drill or whatever else.[1] Ms Elm emphasised the way, in her training, they were taught that in massaging the thigh, you keep off the inner side at the top. Ms Poplar on the other hand had been trained by a man who insisted that you do the whole lot, otherwise it was just polishing the skin. She did add that it was an elderly man. Ms Elm also mentioned that she did have other cases and problems in mind but was afraid of over-balancing the seminar with them, although it was not altogether clear why.

What Ms Poplar's case did bring out is how disturbing it is if the normal barriers and inhibitions are crashed through. Ms Sycamore spoke of how disturbing it was to realise suddenly just how intimate some of the things are that you do. It would not be possible to go on with the work if one maintained a full awareness of the possibilities for sexual excitement at the same time. I emphasised that it was not only a matter of sexual titillation and excitement that had to be suppressed, but also anxieties about the body and its decay that had to be suppressed. We could see that some sort of suppression was often necessary, to enable you to go on with the work, but suppression and blindness carried its own disturbance, and paralysis and distortion of thought.

Note
1 See session on 31st January, 1973.

Thirty-eighth meeting — Wednesday, 14th March, 1973

Case 62 (Ms Beech) — follow-up
Continues from her last report. Since then two quite striking developments. After four further unavailing attempts to see the physical medicine specialist, Ms Beech went to speak to her superintendent about it and this caused an almighty row in front of four other physiotherapists. It was, perhaps, the last straw in a bad week for the superintendent, but the balloon went up and acrimony flew about. The centre of the matter appears to have been this woman telling Ms Beech that the doctor's time was worth much more than hers and Ms Beech standing her ground. Ms Beech was also aware that this woman is volatile and would possibly lose her temper and she had decided beforehand that she was not going to lose hers — and in this, she succeeded. Now Ms Beech has taken up her new position, in a more remote part of the hospital, and relations were still sufficiently bad for the superintendent to send the deputy over to escort Ms Beech into position. Nevertheless, to her surprise, there have been important changes in that she (Ms Beech) has been attached to one physical medicine specialist's clinics, in order that they can get to know each other in a realistic way. Secondly, *he* has been induced to allocate one half-hour each week, as being a time when physiotherapists can consult with him. This has already started, and promises to work well.

With regard to the patient, the second striking development. She had been referred for electro-myography and had then seen the ENT surgeon with the results. He had told her there didn't appear to be any progress.

165

Somehow, when she reported this to Ms Beech, Ms Beech felt strengthened and enabled to take up the prognosis more honestly and straightforwardly. She took the woman in hand and firmly encouraged her that she had better think now in terms of months rather than days. Actually, this detailed exposition of what she said came out only right at the end of the discussion. The woman responded by revealing that the physical medicine doctor had in fact not said anything at all about the alleged guarantee of recovery. She appears to have no recollection of having even thought that he did.

Most of our discussion was around the nature of this collusion between women, to make themselves into pseudo-feminine objects, doormats, while (allegedly) the men treat them in some high and mighty way. For me, this linked with the collusion between Ms Beech and the patient to be mismanaged and maltreated, by incredible remarks from the doctor. What impressed me was the way the row amongst the women enables a more realistic view of the man to emerge. Ms Beech's position this week is utterly different from last week and she now appears to have a quite genial and optimistic view of this chap, whereas he did sound pretty impossible last week.

I tried also to get on to the concreteness[1] around this — specific beliefs attaching to the question of whether you do or do not possess a penis. Thence the question of substitutes and equivalents like machinery, electromyograms and so forth.[2] When Ms Beech feels stiffened by an EMG (electromyogram report) she may behave like a new woman.

Ms Teak emphasised the more general sense that patients (apart from engineers!) tend to be extraordinarily accepting and uncurious in the face of nonsensical treatments. I took this as a reminder that this problem of pathological passivity, and the travesty of femininity, is not a problem confined to women. Of course many men behave in exactly the same way, and invite good or bad omnipotent behaviour, from strong male figures — or strong female ones! There was a further digression into the question of women doctors and what they are like, but I tried to re-focus matters around the particular problems of being a woman in what is largely a woman's profession, somewhat under the thumb of men. The threat of things getting worse, with every treatment being confined to prescription by a doctor, is arousing militant rebellion. The superintendent has actually, since the row last week, deputed Ms Beech to take part in some representation that is being made there in her hospital.

Case 64 (Ms Lime)

She wished to note some anxieties about locum work she will be undertaking during the next few months in ante-natal and post-natal clinics or wards at her present hospital, where she works part-time. (She also does classes at home for the National Childbirth Trust.) There are various complaints: Ms Lime is isolated there; her work is blurred indistinguishably from that of a nurse which is resented on both sides; she is allowed excellent access and indeed mixes in with nursing procedures in the labour ward, in great contrast with the ante-natal and post-natal situations. Aside from the general trouble of having to work and fit into a style which she disapproves of, a style in which any sort of human interchange of communications is militated against, the classes are very much classes to teach exercises and physical procedures but not to encourage talk.

This leads to the next and really major problem — that there is an embargo on the physiotherapist 'answering any questions'. Once a physiotherapist

166

told a woman to go home and not worry when she had reported some slight bleeding and in fact she and the baby nearly died of an ante-partum haemorrhage. Following this disaster the physiotherapist is now not allowed to arrogate to herself any midwifery knowledge at all and no questions may be asked or answered. This directly relates to the problem of Ms Beech and the first case — the question of when the physiotherapist is licensed and indeed in duty bound, to speak out from her knowledge. When, by contrast, does she have to realise or pretend that she is 'only a layman'?

This led on to further discussions about the magic of white coats and the responsibilities which go with wearing them — and thence I reminded them of this same concrete question, where the white coat, the EMG etc, stand for something like a definite physical appendage, linked in many people's minds with a sort of magic penis. It does seem to be an enormous, world-shaking departure for Ms Lime *to dare* to take her classes without a white coat — and indeed she does not dare do it in the hospital, only in her own home.

Notes

1 The development here concerns our understanding of the way confidence, trust, optimism and pessimism, attitudes regarding status, prestige and skill — all these apparently abstract considerations may be locked to the most banal physical considerations. People *do* 'believe in' the magic of uniforms and titles; a doctor can indeed feel different with a stethoscope around his neck; a physiotherapist can feel an expert amongst experts when she holds an electromyography report in her hand. At depth, these appendages can carry a charge from the magical aura that we all attach to the sexual objects that excite us. If the *latent* beliefs suggested here appear to be of fatuous naïveté, it must be remembered that we are constantly confronted by medical behaviour and hospital habits of such astounding and *manifest* inappropriateness that only an Alice in Wonderland type of thinking can explain it.

2 See also the conclusion to Ms Lime's case following.

Thirty-ninth meeting — Wednesday, 21st March, 1973

Case 65 (Ms Sycamore)

A girl of 14 who appears to have an hysterical disorder on one knee. Incredibly, two years ago the surgeons removed her patella and, after further messing about, (EUAs and MUAs etc) they have now referred her to the physiotherapy department. The problem is that there does not appear to be any self-respecting notion of physiotherapy for a hysterical or 'functional' disorder. Instead, there is a thin attempt to rationalise the referral in some physical terms and, correspondingly, the physiotherapists feel insulted and exploited. We then get a lot of posturing behind talk about 'a queue of more deserving people who urgently need attention'. Or, on the other hand, 'if it is psychological' immediate thoughts of psychiatrists, social workers etc. The fact is that a large proportion of their work is covertly of this sort. I would have thought that it might make matters easier if it were overt. Nobody but myself really expressed the sense of outrage anyway about the mutilation of this girl's leg by the surgeon.

Case 6 (Ms Oak) – follow-up

Another of her rather rambling presentations which I find hard to get hold of. This is the case formerly treated by Ms Ash and reported here – the patient who had been a physiotherapist many years ago and now has an unmanageable variety of aches and pains. Whenever there is a question of instructing her in exercises she proceeds to do them at tremendous speed and is always a step or two ahead of the physiotherapist who is supposed to be treating her. Within this setting, there are unfathomable problems of locating quite what the disorder is, or its nature. The assumption appears to be that it is hysterical too, but there is some protest, especially from Ms Teak. There is a feeling that this woman has not really been thoroughly investigated by competent people, especially by somebody specialising in backs, but she has now been through the departments of two teaching hospitals.

Fortieth meeting – Wednesday, 28th March, 1973

Case 62 (Ms Beech) – follow-up

The doctor in her recent case now turns out to be a 'terribly nice guy'. He is young, approachable, keen for change and is 'totally oblivious of the protection racket' going on around him. Ms Beech is delighted with all this and everyone is suitably impressed at the way things have changed. However, he is still in ignorance of the barriers around him. As a result of Ms Beech's efforts access is now improved and there is a regular time for physiotherapists to come and see him, but we are not at all sure whether the basic state of affairs, ie of a nice guy surrounded by a barrier of embattled women, is any different. Ms Beech does not feel she could go through the same experience again.[1]

Case 66 (Ms Poplar)

Frankly brought as the need to discharge what she has on her mind and 'not really a physio case at all'. Travelling to work this morning there was a woman collapsed on the platform of a tube station and nobody doing much. Ms Poplar was joined by a trainee nurse and between them they gave cardiac massage and mouth-to-mouth breathing which 'was really working'. She gave a dramatic description of how horrible it all was but, nevertheless, she was able to get on with it and saw the pupils dilate and contract with each cardiac thrust and colour returned. But the only railway official was sceptical, unhelpful and slow and it was 25 minutes, on her watch, before an ambulance appeared. She was bitterly distraught and upset by this and began to cry in the seminar at the thought. She had sent somebody else off to hurry up the ambulance and to ask for a resuscitation equipment ambulance, which she knew to exist in the district. The ambulance drivers finally did trundle the patient upstairs, trying to continue the cardiac massage as they went. There was no sucker and no airway until they produced one, with which they bashed a couple of teeth down her throat. Ms Poplar had to retrieve the airway which was not working and found the two teeth embedded in the end. They got her into the ambulance but she appeared to be dead on arrival at hospital. At hospital the difference and the efficiency were highly impressive and she has nothing but praise for the speed and skill with which they got on with it there: and they continued trying for about half an hour. At one point they gave up but she persuaded them to have another go. But it was of no avail. She was very

168

impressed by the combination of efficiency and detached uninvolvement, that enabled them to joke good-humouredly with her, while in no way reducing their attention and effort. In contrast, she found herself, outside her white coat, involved in a way that astonished her.

I was struck by a number of things. Firstly the continued need for God Almighty, for miracle workers, and this is involved in the collusion of women to set up the man as the big white chief.

Secondly there is the need to maintain this sense of what miracles one could only do if only, eg if only the men were more competent or facilities were better, or if one had a sucker or a defibrilator, etc.

This led on to a discussion about how the physiotherapist should behave, when directed to continue with a stupid and futile treatment. Ms Teak's discussion had led to some notion of possible firm and polite behaviour, as a physiotherapist, which would not be the same thing as becoming lost in a rebellious altercation. But what was also exposed was the contrast between the work of the physiotherapist (and, I realise, psychiatrist!) whose work is hardly ever life-saving and the surgeon whose work appears, so often, to be dramatically life-saving. While we know that the reality of the surgeon's work may be very much more humdrum, the difference does remain and this is somehow linked with *our* preoccupation with miracles, people behaving like God and our need for them to do so.[2]

(Behind all this again is the ever-with-us question of Ms Poplar's sister with the inoperable tumour.)

Case 67 (Ms Oak)

Again, we did not allow enough time for it and she took the remaining 20 minutes in monologue. It was interesting and appeared to show certain considerable development on her part, but still in the form of an uninterruptable and shapeless story. This is a patient who is being treated for a stiff and painful neck, for which there is probably no organic cause. She has had MUAs[3] before and is in for another one. It appears to have made no difference — as expected — but it was confirmed that, under anaesthetic, mobility was normal.[4] Ms Oak has found herself gently exploring this woman's experience with her, including some mention of her husband's violence, putting his hands round her neck (ie where the symptoms are) and threatening to strangle her. Ms Oak's line has been a rather timid exploration, punctuated by the notion that 'perhaps you might tell the doctor that when you see him'.[5]

Notes

1 We missed the seriousness of this. Ms Beech never returned to the seminar after this week. She wrote to say she found the emotional strain too much.

2 The point here is that whereas surgeons and physicians can readily find dramatic satisfaction in their work and can enjoy an ambience of life-saving and magic in the course of their daily activities, physiotherapists may carry more of the grinding chronic conditions, while their treatments are slow and of doubtful efficacy. This means a job involving anxiety — envying and idealising the imagined facile joys of being a surgeon.

3 Manipulation under anaesthetic.

4 ie implying that the disability involves muscular spasm and is possibly of psychological origin.

5 This note does not do justice to the struggle going on. Members of the

Tavistock GP and Allied Professional Workshop studying a transcript of this session later were impressed at the distance this physiotherapist had covered. We have the case of a woman, presenting with a pain in the neck (!), stuck in a regime of futile treatments (involving, *inter alia*, general anaesthetics — which are not altogether without danger) that enable her real problems to persist unregarded. She has a violent husband and a son who attempted suicide. The professional problem for the seminar is to evolve styles of work that enable the physiotherapist to develop her skill in eliciting crucial information and enlarging insight, yet avoiding becoming saddled with unmanageable burdens.

Forty-first meeting — Wednesday, 4th April, 1973

Case 58 (Ms Sycamore) — follow-up

Briefly, a middle-aged woman who had a below-knee amputation for cellulitis with severe septicaemia — nearly fatal before the operation. She had been in an intensive care unit for a month or more after the operation and has been an in-patient since October — five or six months. She had previously reported the dreadfully slow progress of physiotherapy against the fixed flexion of the knee and the total wastage of the quadriceps muscles. Since then, there has been some improvement, only following MUAs, which have been done now three times. She is flat out for several days after each anaesthetic, in a way that is rather strange. Otherwise, she is a somewhat excitable woman.

The present situation is that the surgeon, having been in the USA since last autumn, has now returned and suggested discharge home. Home is in Bromley and the proposal is that she be brought up by transport for daily physiotherapy. Ms Sycamore notices a strange state of excitement from the patient and connects this more with the return of the surgeon than with the discharge impending. She has been going home for weekends anyway for a considerable time, living with her married sister and brother-in-law.

Ms Sycamore recalls our previous discussion and a sense that feelings about the surgeon, who had performed the amputation, might be a very important factor in this woman's reactions. Ms Sycamore doesn't really know quite what to say, or where to go from here. There seems to be something rather unrealistic about the idea that the woman will attend from Bromley, each day, and a sense of clinging to unrealities hangs about the case. Ms Sycamore speaks wistfully about the possibility of another MUA, instead of taking a businesslike realistic line if (as is the case) she thinks it is the best thing to do and has been productive so far. Actually, my impression is that she shares in the patient's unrealistic and wistful feelings to do with restoring the leg, or something of that sort, and hence the strained reaction to each anaesthetic, as if it is an echo of the original operation, which it should have reversed.

As a shot in the dark, I asked what happened to the amputated leg and this did reveal a striking blank. It was quite hard for Ms Sycamore to realise that, eventually, the limb would probably have been incinerated; but she did, in fact, recall a conversation with the patient in which they had discussed some tests that had been done on the removed part. This was supposed to have been to find out the cause of the problem, but no real information did emerge.

170

Case 68 (Ms Teak)

This started around generalities but really seemed to be about pain and the management of one or two cases of depression after back operations.[1] The patients continue to be nurses, for the most part, and this is another curious story in itself. She had had a discussion/argument with a young surgeon although, when she reproduced it, it was impossible for us to see really what their difference was. He had told her that the patient should be given a straight account of what had happened and what they might expect and that she 'was not to give them a pat on the back'. She does not really see herself as actually giving pats on the back, or empty encouragement, so the difficulty is rather hard to focus. It seems to include at least two questions: (1) the question of whose responsibility is it to explain to people what they are to expect? (2) what is the attitude to pain and what is the physiotherapist's responsibility in the management?

What struck me was that while there were subtle discussions of how people should be prepared for pain, or managed through it, and general expectations that if only the right attitude is taken up the pain will be bearable, what was strikingly missing was any notion of the use of analgesics. The general expectation was that somehow, by magic, the pain ought to go away if only you get the right frame of mind. In other words, we are facing the ease with which other people's pain can be denied. There was some discussion of the distinction between pain and distress — the question of what are the additional factors which turn pain into unbearable distress — feelings about whether it can be avoided. There is some indication that when the analgesics are quite clearly available it is possible for the patient to decline them, whereas they get angry and miserable when drugs are not available until sister does her round, or the houseman comes in, or whatever.

Note
1 A few weeks previously this very experienced physiotherapist had registered her personal impression that every back operation is followed by a reaction of depression.

Forty-second meeting — Wednesday, 11th April, 1973

Case 6 (Ms Oak) — follow-up

This is reported, mainly to add another detail to the case she inherited from Ms Ash, but it leaves us in the same ill-defined area as before. The new point is that Ms Oak had got this woman patient (the ex-physiotherapist) to make certain movements at the shoulder, as part of the effort to improve posture. As a result, Ms Oak gets a sardonic humorous message back from the consultant, when they next meet, to say that Ms Oak now appears to have produced fresh symptoms in that shoulder, where there were none before. It is clear that no one thinks there is any physical basis for this woman's aches and pains. We are now getting to have a sense that they move around on invitation. Meanwhile, Ms Oak is ploughing on very half-heartedly with posture. She is also getting the patient to reduce weight and has indeed got nine pounds off her. It also emerges that there is a 13-year-old daughter with asthma. Ms Lime urges the possibility of a course of relaxation, if it could be combined with the opportunity to talk. There is fresh rumination about the possibility of other investigations, back investigations etc, although this ground has been gone over many times. The problem seems to be to get this physiotherapist out of the clutches of other physiotherapists and doctors, and towards some sort of psychological help. Nobody was sure. Another difficulty is that, as with the shoulder, she may be liable to develop fresh symptoms wherever you look whether it be in her bones or in her mind.

Case 58 (Ms Sycamore) – follow-up
Following last week (the lady with the below-knee amputation), she did ask for another MUA, which was duly performed. The benefit seems to have been somewhat marginal and they appear to be now near the limits of bony deformity so there is only the remaining question of stabilising this recent gain of a few degrees.

Simultaneously, Ms Sycamore had discovered within herself, the ability to get in touch with the doctors. She is now seeing them, has shown a new Registrar around the department and is impressed with the change this represents in herself, rather than in them. Has there been the same clinging to some faulty relationship as there was, in the patient, a clinging to the bad leg, and to the hospital?

The patient is due to go home at Easter and there is a question of what use should be made of the remaining week and a half. Right at the end, we discover that this woman may have exaggerated hopes of her 'final' prosthesis when it comes – she walks very well with a pylon at the moment but has exaggerated hopes of doing Greek dancing and heaven knows what when her artificial limb arrives. There is some doubt as to whether she has had a really good look at one – but then the cat gets out of the bag: neither have most of the members of the seminar! Surprisingly, it is all very much at the level of 'having seen one once' in particular patients some time ago – maybe. This scotoma is parallel with the difficulty in seeing the amputated limb, in the mind's eye, and having any idea what becomes of it. The patient is, at this moment, 'flat out' as usual, after the MUA.

Case 63 (Ms Poplar) – follow-up
This is the 'obscene' woman – the 'old woman of at least 43' who was behaving 'like a promiscuous 16-year-old'. During the last discussion, Ms Poplar felt herself dislodged from a position in which she was trying to address the woman as someone her mother's age, while struggling inwardly with a quite different view. She changed her tactic and took a much firmer line that this woman must now get on her feet and get a job and behave like a grown-up, expressing a firm conviction that she would be perfectly able to do so and that she could not require Ms Poplar to tell her how to find a job, or rooms, etc. Ms Poplar promised her two more weekly appointments 'before the chop', although holding out a vague prospect that she could return if necessary, but the conviction is that it would not be necessary.

The woman did not turn up for either appointment but came a week later. Ms Poplar jumped on her with the information that her place had been taken and that she (Ms Poplar) could not see her, only to be thoroughly wrong-footed. The patient announced that she had not come for treatment but merely to thank Ms Poplar for all her help and to say that she had now got a job cleaning theatres, which is what she had wanted. (We are reminded that this woman seeks a career in the theatre and is content, meantime, to act as a cleaner in one, with hopeful talk of being 'discovered' one day.)

We discussed the question of whether Ms Poplar had been demoting or up-grading the patient. She had thought she was down-grading her into a little girl whom she could boss about and she is puzzled at the result. Some people felt that there was an up-grading to the role of an adult woman to whom a sexual life is permitted, instead of being viewed as a geriatric menopausal woman, who should behave like Ms Poplar's mother is pictured as doing, or, more probably, her grandmother. We further note that whether it be up-grading or down-grading, there is the discovery of strength in the physiotherapist – that a patient is liable to respond, sometimes, as if you are a magician, capable of bestowing decrepitude or youth, merely by the way you view the patient – rather like living up to expectations.

A further point – Ms Poplar emphasised that what really seemed to her unforgiveable in a middle-aged woman were the stupidities, like setting fire to her wastepaper basket, rather than the sexualities. Everybody laughed at the notion that they had missed out on the permissive opportunities – that at 16 they might have been free to be promiscuous and light fires. We note that the notion of danger becomes replaced by notions of private moralities and rules.

Forty-third meeting – Wednesday, 9th May, 1973

I began by telling them that I had received a letter from Ms Beech saying that she now found Wednesdays too difficult and that I had written back to remonstrate.

Ms Teak reported – perhaps to reassure us that it is all worth while – that there is considerable interest in the work of the seminar at her hospital. People always ask about it (including senior nursing staff) and have said how useful they think it might be for all of them to have a seminar of this sort. I said we had better do something to justify this optimism.

Case 58 (Ms Sycamore) – follow-up
Her lady with the below-knee amputation has now been discharged and the main point is the enormous relief Ms Sycamore feels. On her instigation, one more MUA was performed prior to discharge and the bony limit of mobilisation has now been reached. The severe reaction to anaesthetics had previously been noted but this one surpassed the others.

Ms Sycamore was also concerned at the degree of disappointment experienced by this patient following a visit to Roehampton for the fitting of an artificial limb. She had warned her that very little might be achieved on this visit and that it might prove difficult, at first, to stand up on the new limb, let alone dance around with it, which seemed to be the patient's expectation. In spite of these explanations and warnings, there was a distinctly depressed reaction. There was quite a long discussion about this problem of patients who 'don't get the message', however much effort you put into explanations and warnings. It was recognised that there must be a serious failure to engage with the real problem when this happens and that, on our side, there is also some failure to 'get the message' if we continue to repeat ourselves in a way that is manifestly inappropriate and unsuccessful. In course of this topic, more information about this patient came out. It seems there is a 17-year history of trouble with this leg which had been fractured in childhood. There has also been a hysterectomy.

Interestingly, the present point at issue, that Ms Sycamore failed 'to get across', hinges on the same issue about which the case was first presented to us. This is the problem of straightening the knee and, following the last MUA, Ms Sycamore has been trying to convey, frankly and firmly, that the

173

knee is now as straight as it is ever going to get. (At first, Ms Sycamore was at war with the doctors because they expected her to achieve the impossible , in straightening this knee.) Many of the other difficulties, physical as well as psychological, stem from the need to face this fact. There is an important distinction between cases where you get the feedback that tells you that the patient did not register your messages and instructions — as distinct from the many cases where you never realise that this has happened. Ms Lime urges the value of domiciliary treatment, in this connection. It is possible to verify whether things have been understood or not, with your own eyes.

I was inclined to re-emphasise that this is a two-way problem. It is equally a problem of the extraordinary ability of medical people, including physiotherapists, to fail to hear messages that patients tell us again and again, in their own way — messages about their anxieties, messages that the treatment is not going to work, messages that their expectations are wildly unrealistic and so on. Yet we manage to be repeatedly outraged when things turn out exactly the way we have been warned.

Case 69 (Ms Teak)
This follows directly and was stirred by the previous discussion. This is a man who has had a laminectomy and spinal fusion and who drives everybody beyond the limits of tolerance by his repetition of the same questions, expressing his anxiety about his operation, prognosis etc. All the explanations in the world did not seem to touch his anxiety. Eventually, Ms Teak had it out with him, whereupon he said that really it was his wife who was anxious and kept on at him and they did not know how she would manage with him and the three children when he came home. How far this was true is uncertain but this change of tack produced a considerable abatement of his pressure. Incidentally, this led to some discussion of the advice to 'take care of yourself' which is one of the more useless and disturbing injunctions that we give our victims.

Case 61 (Ms Oak) — follow-up
This is the man with the cerebral tumour who wanted to use a walking stick instead of a tripod. He has now died at home. Ms Oak had some discussion with the wife in the meantime which has clarified certain aspects of the case. It seems that the wife was given the true diagnosis some time ago and arranged that she would, herself, impart the truth to her husband at home. She did this. However, he survived 'beyond his allotted time' and there was a feeling that this contributed to the unrealistic phase, during which he behaved as if he was going to get better and better. It was as if the doctors had been proved wrong, for a time.

Case 70 (Ms Oak)
A woman of about 38 is admitted with acute rheumatoid arthritis. In the routine way, the physiotherapist is called in and fixes up splints, and attends to making the patient comfortable in a good position. Then, over the next week, tests come back and they all slowly realise that this is a full-blown case of hysteria that has fooled them. The tests are all normal. The severe pain is not due to any detectable physical lesion and the swollen joints, noticed on first examination, turn out to be knobbly knees in a thin woman.

She is a gym teacher and Ms Oak elicits the fact that she is jaded with it, but does not really find out much else. It is striking that, unlike most hysterics, this woman does not get herself disliked and she seems to be distinctly compliant. She did lead the nurses quite a dance, with her needs,

174

but everybody else finds her very nice. She has been transferred to the psychiatric ward and has gone, like a lamb, without a murmur. Ms Oak continues to visit her there and has continued to provide her attentions, as a physiotherapist, to help make her comfortable and contented — even though it is no longer a case of treating rheumatoid arthritis. This seems to be in keeping with this pattern of a patient who remains on good terms with everybody and fits in.

It is also most unusual the way she has been bundled off to the psychiatric ward. The psychiatrist was called in by the physical medicine consultant, as soon as he realised the nature of the condition. This is in contrast to the more usual pattern of events, whereby investigations proliferate and the turning over of stones continues until everybody is sick of it. In this case, the psychiatrist was called in immediately and took the patient into his ward forthwith.

Forty-fourth meeting — Wednesday, 16th May, 1973

Ms Teak was talking about patients who are not successfully reassured by pre-operative chats but, above all, she was talking about her tendency to feel guilty and responsible for anything that goes wrong with a patient's treatment, whether it is her fault or not — or indeed whether it is anybody's fault.

Cases 71 and 72 (Ms Teak)
There were two examples. One Mr Khan, a likeable Indian sailor who had injured a knee in Lisbon, had treatment and an infected haematoma, eventually treated at the — Hospital, where he is now having a quadriceps transplant, a distinctly unusual operation. This seems not to have gone very well and hence the soul-searchings as to responsibility and wondering whether the physiotherapy pulled the wound open, necessitating skin graft. General agreement that 'no one is responsible'.

The other case is a woman who had a total replacement of hip joint and who then was unwisely got out of bed and not helped back by a nurse. Ms Teak has some qualms as to whether she should have warned the woman against any such possibility. The result was a re-dislocation of the repaired joint but it was discovered that the whole thing was extremely unstable: the dislocation was an unusual one in the anterior direction owing to some unusual shape of the joint. Hence, again, the agreement that nobody is to blame but the patient has loudly and understandably complained about the nurse to Ms Teak.

There was some discussion about underlying feelings, eg grandiose wishes to take on responsibility for everything, secret triumph over people who are actually responsible and do the wrong thing (covered by this show of self-accusation). The reactions include problems of loyalty, idealisation of the group to which one belongs, etc. There is also the problem of susceptibility to patients who thrive on playing people off and driving in wedges. There is the temptation to be 'the only person who understands' and so on.

Case 73 (Ms Lime)
In association to all this, Ms Lime mentioned a number of situations that she encounters in hospital, fragmentary aspects of general problems — and hard for me to judge whether this is by way of illumination or, on the

contrary, whether it represents a systematic superficiality. She particularly mentioned the case of the woman who has absorbable sutures in the perineum, after an episiotomy, and has been told by the woman doctor that they will not need to be taken out. This is perfectly true and the buried part of the sutures is absorbed but the suture ends remaining on the surface do often have to be removed. So far as the patient is concerned, this amounts to a betrayal of promises. Ms Lime, as the person in between, and as a good listener, tends to get told; but then what is *her* resposnibility and who should *she* tell?

Case 74 (Ms Yew)
Ms Yew was drawn into mentioning an episode a year ago, when she had accidentally broken a child's leg. The child suffers from some rare and peculiar disease and it was really a pathological fracture. She was following instructions to continue a routine of exercises that the duty physiotherapist was supposed to come in and do. So she did it during her tour of duty and reported the unusual mobility of the joint that appeared to follow. It only emerged some hours later that the fracture had occurred unbeknown to herself and to the little boy. Again, obviously not 'her fault', but what about all the feelings generated in herself and around and about?

Forty-fifth meeting — Wednesday, 23rd May, 1973

Case 72 (Ms Teak) — follow-up
The lady with the total hip replacement which dislocated. At last, with much anxiety on both sides, they got her up yesterday, without mishap. The discussion really was around the content and management of this 'anxiety on both sides'. It is clear that this was circumscribed around the more obvious anxiety, as to whether it would go wrong again and the discussion of this was done as a once-off affair by the registrar with the patient, last week. The present policy becomes one of any further anxiety remaining unspoken and a general atmosphere of whistling in the dark. Ms Yew is totally blank and silent and Ms Lime is aware, clearly enough, that she would handle it more intuitively or impulsively, but nobody finds it possible to enlarge or open the question of the issues involved, systematically. Ms Lime is indeed concerned that her own 'method' is so dependent on the feeling of the moment. I tried to lead this trio through some sense of what you might run into if you open this up and what might be the purpose of so doing.

The first thought in Ms Teak's mind (which she thought was my worry) was the question of litigation and recrimination. This led, by free-association, to her description of how she herself had had a swab left inside her following an operation and she mentioned some of the factors in her own mind, for and against litigation at that time, eg the pressure of relatives for litigation; and her own wish for peace and quiet in her professional life, against it. This clarified certain possible directions but, especially the general one, namely, that if you push your enquiries with somebody, you are likely to end up in a more personal realm than you may have intended. Thus with Ms Teak. With the patient, we might land in unexpected territory, about her relations with her family and what they feel about her and her anxieties about the nature of the condition etc.

Case 75 (Ms Yew)
Presented against all the tide of her inclination to blank everything off and

176

see everything as 'just normal'. We did agree that being in hospital altogether can never be 'just normal'. She came up with a case, 'not my own case' (which seems to be a recurrent thing, this business of presenting only cases that are not her own). There was some passing mention of the problem of a boy who is moderately disabled, due to congenital malformations resulting from maternal rubella in pregnancy. The boy complains that it is 'not my fault' and, transparently, feels that it is mother's fault or somebody's fault.

Case 76 (Ms Yew)
However, the case more deliberately presented is of another child, who appears to have a minimal physical disability, undiagnosed moreover, but with some peculiar psychological problem. He was, apparently, hit by a car but got up and ran away. Whether following this or coincidentally, he has a peculiar gait, with rather floppy feet, but no other abnormal physical signs. Apparently, he crawls around the house at home, rather than walking and, so far as home is concerned, is severely disabled. He is an only child, It is known that the father is an alcoholic and allegedly takes no interest. The general diagnosis at the hospital is that nothing much can be done until, if, and when, something better develops at home. Meantime, the aim is for the hospital, (ie the physiotherapists) to provide whatever they can, as support. So he comes to the physiotherapy department and charges round the gym at great speed most of the time and Ms Yew could do nothing particular with him. There are hints of feeble and futile conversations with mother but it is equally futile to try to get past Ms Yew's own stance. I did expose the dilemma with which we are faced — that there is something pretty drastically wrong with either her hospital, or Ms Yew, or both, to explain this massively blocked absence of any healthy curiosity about their patients, or any ability to think about them. Obviously (I did not say this), the present picture has something to do with Ms Yew having been more or less sent by them and representing a superficial co-operation which covers the terrified obstinate fear of learning anything that would disturb.

Forty-sixth meeting — Wednesday, 30th May, 1973

Case 70 (Ms Oak) — follow-up
The gym teacher with rheumatoid arthritis (?), (see session on 28th March, 1973), which turned out to be hysteria. She has now been fully taken over by the psychiatric department and long-term psychotherapy planned (? started). Ms Oak has been going into that ward anyway and retaining some supportive contact with the patient but her formal connection is now finished. Ms Oak judges that without her initiative the case would have dragged on with abortive physiotherapy for some considerable time and that probably the seminar helped her to be more business-like about it.

Case 72 (Ms Teak) — follow-up
The case of the total hip replacement which dislocated. Since the seminar told her that she had blocked the patient from the chance of expressing her anxieties about getting up, she decided to reform. During a 'mini-round' with the Registrar she told him the woman was worried and asked him to reassure her, which he did, in telling her that there was no more chance of her hip dislocating than anybody else's. There is considerable

uncertainty whether any distinction was made, in this respect, between normal hips and plastic ones, and one continues to get the atmosphere of whistling in the dark a bit. It also emerged late in the discussion that Ms Teak herself was rather astonished by this and has been convinced, only with some difficulty, that things might be as good as that. However, it seems that a plastic hip tends to stabilise as time goes on, and each day gained is a step to that end. We discussed the choice of the Registrar, rather than doing it herself, and this is now seen as connected with her own grave doubts, which the Registrar evidently did not have, or at any rate did not voice. Any notions from last week of exposing herself to any larger anxieties of a personal kind, lying behind this, were totally forgotten. The only question to be admitted as worthy of discussion is whether the hip will or will not dislocate again. Ms Teak felt rather niggled by me, bridling somewhat, but remaining firmly good-humoured. I tried to re-establish the notion that we were exposing options, possibilities and a sense of where it might take you, *if* you follow certain lines — rather than advocating that anybody should do so. There may be clear indications for not doing so.

Case 77 (Ms Teak)

A man she describes as batty and whom she maintains everybody else finds batty, too. It is impossible to get further with what she means except that the man is incomprehensible and uncomprehending. He has had a spinal fusion and has a very bad hip too, which has not been done yet. She is afraid that he will muck the whole thing up by bending his back. Ms Sycamore tried to press her into really examining what her anxieties were, what exactly she envisaged happening, but was firmly blocked on this with the reiteration of general notions about failed operations, fusions 'not working', and so on. We touched on general questions about why a patient might behave in this relentlessly blind-to-danger way, including the effort to project anxiety into everybody else.[1] Ms Sycamore had mentioned a case where she has transferred her anxiety by transferring the patient to somebody else; and this gave me the lead on that one.

Case 64 (Ms Lime) — follow-up

Really regarding her situation about ante-natal training classes in her hospital, where she is rather blocked by the midwives but is instituting some research approach via the gynaecologist and via a college of London University. She has been warned off approaching the psychiatrists.[2]

Notes

1 The point here is that behaviour which appears blithely to disregard risk may be serving to free the subject himself from anxiety, whilst transposing it into someone else, who may (hopefully) be better able to deal with it.
2 Hospital politics!

Forty-seventh meeting — Wednesday, 6th June, 1973

A day of open discussion about the profession of physiotherapy rather than presentation of cases.

As I arrived, Ms Sycamore had just announced that she is expecting a baby in the late summer. She will be with us until the seminar is due to stop at the end of term, but will then be withdrawing from physiotherapy — for a substantial time at any rate. Although, in a sense, it was transparent that this released much comment and dissatisfaction from the others, it was not until the last bit of the seminar that a real sense of the dynamic emerged.

At first, the discussion seemed to spring from Ms Elm's sense of dissatisfaction and disillusion — and her plans to leave physiotherapy whenever she can find something else suitable. There is the usual basic complaint of being over-trained and under-valued and underpaid. She would like work where she would be required to exert and stretch herself, and to be paid accordingly. There is no reward for extra effort in the present set-up. As in other branches of the paramedical professions, there is financial pressure to move over to the teaching side, where there is slightly more pay, but even less satisfaction in the work.

This led to many sour thoughts about training of physiotherapists, the stupidity of the curriculum and the exams, the failure of teachers to be taught how to teach. Quite a number of remarks were made acknowledging the reasonably steady improvement in this sort of thing as the years go by, but the overwhelming balance of feeling was that the training they had was poor and that the training the youngsters are now getting is not much better.

Of course, this had a lot to do with the wish to be better trained to handle psychological problems and the emotional aspects of their work. Somehow linked with this, there was also painful doubt as to the rationale of most physiotherapy and a painful sense of its unproven value. They may have a lively sense of doing valuable work much of the time, but there is still a painful sense that the things they do may often be concessions to ritual and ceremony, more than anything else. Thence, all mixed up with sporadic complaints about the elders/matriarchs of the profession, there was a discussion about teaching.

Firstly, there was the feeling of regret at losing the satisfaction of working directly with patients. Supposedly, this would be compensated by the interest of working with the students, but this just does not materialise. They find it frustrating to hand the patients over, especially if it means watching things being done awkwardly. Moreover, teaching seems to involve quite a bit of demonstration on students, involving touching them, massaging them, etc. Ms Elm has discovered waves of revulsion in herself from this, nasty thoughts wondering what the students suspect of her sexuality!

One of our rare discussions about massage and touching ensued. The emphasis was mainly on anxiety and distaste about this work, but Ms Lime also brought out the other side — the resistance that has to be overcome amongst colleagues if you do wish to use massage as a regular technique. An ostensible objection is that it takes up too much time, the department cannot afford so much one-to-one work. However, they seemed to agree that other varieties of touching, for example in connection with chests (breathing exercises, postural drainage, etc) did not seem to carry the same anxiety for them, or question from anybody else.

Another discussion was about uniforms, again stemming mainly from Ms Elm. At first the emphasis seemed entirely to be on resentment of being put in a uniform and scorn of a profession and a system that forces this on you. There is a tremendous wish to appear, on the job, as oneself and not as somebody-in-a-white-coat or somebody in a mysterious hierarchical structure — a red-belt or a green-belt or whatever.

This partly arose in a context of envy of younger sisters and other friends who had gone into other professions and were doing very nicely thank you

179

very much (without all these petty restrictions). This seemed to me to be getting out of touch with reality and there was swift agreement when I reminded them of the frequent relief at being in a white coat (eg Ms Elm herself was glad of her white coat when her private patient's grown-up son wanted her to massage his back and she had some difficulty in remaining in charge[1]). (We could also contrast this with the episode of Ms Poplar without her white coat in the underground station.[2]) Of course, if there is a secure professional sense internally and you are *not* before the patient simply as yourself, with all your own impulses undisguised, then it may be quite possible to dispense with uniforms and, thereby, gain flexibility and intimacy. In any case, it is clear that physiotherapists have to struggle with distasteful and disturbing feelings within themselves, especially about physical contact with patients and this is indeed a strange moment to be proposing a gay abandon of uniforms and of inhibitions. Admittedly this was not strictly being proposed.

From further grumbling — and discussion of the extensive dissatisfaction in the profession, the rapid turnover of staff, even in departments which are considered to be enlightened and pleasant — I thought we were up against the problem of anxiety and gloom built into the work by its involvement with age and disease. This brought some clarification of a sense of difference from doctors and nurses. The latter are felt somehow to be not quite so heavily committed to health and recovery as a 'remedial profession' like physiotherapy. Doctors may have a different professional interest or curiosity in disease process, however much they hope for cures; nurses know that part of their work is going to be caring rather than curing and that they will see people through to the end — although, for that matter, the drop-out rate from nursing is enormous too. Physiotherapists often get lumbered with the care of people for whom nothing else can be done, the aged and decrepit or, worse, the young and crippled — and a lot of the bitterness about the profession, about doctors, about each other, is really displaced from bitterness about the misery of disease and how little you can do about it so much of the time.

Thence, the discussion seemed to wander off again onto envy of people who have better jobs and some preoccupation with people who leave the profession, try something else and come back. For me, this was where the penny dropped and I felt this was about people who leave the profession to have babies and come back. Amongst all the many reasons why these women may wish to be married and have children, there is one very specific hope reposed in having children, which is relevant in this context. This is the sense that having children is a specific antidote to anxieties about illness, age and death. When gloom about illness and death is particularly pressing the idea of having a new baby may become particularly desirable or, indeed, the only worthwhile thing to do in life.

Notes
1 See session on 10th January, 1973.
2 See session on 28th March, 1973.

Forty-eighth meeting — Wednesday, 13th June, 1973

Case 78 (Ms Yew)
The patient is a two-year-old boy suffering from a rare congenital disorder called ?arthrogryphosis. It seems to involve the stiffening of joints and

muscles and, although there is no specific treatment, the management does involve a lot of surgical and physiotherapy attention. The child has had a number of tendon transplants and Ms Yew has recently begun work with this child and his mother.

The problem she presents is that the parents are sueing another hospital where the mother had an operation for appendicitis during pregnancy. They attribute the disease to some mismanagement of the operation and refuse to accept that this congenital disorder is of unknown cause. The mother has asked Ms Yew what she thinks about it — as, indeed, she asks everybody she meets — and Ms Yew describes herself as having 'ducked out of it'. There is the usual exchange based on trying to find out what the surgeon said and, anyway, referring the mother back to him.

We mull this over very slowly, the four of us, as we struggle to get a sense of Ms Yew at work. The mother is described as 'not very chatty' and, later, as a 'bewildered young mum'. We cannot help noticing that these words could apply equally to Ms Yew herself and must have a bearing on her work with this family.

Although it sounds reasonable to defer to the surgeon for the authoritative guidance the family may need about the nature of the arthrogryphosis and its origin, we in the seminar are bound to face up to the fact that Ms Yew describes herself as having 'ducked out of it'. Of course the doctor may supply medical information as, indeed, the solicitor may be consulted for legal information and guidance, but what of the physiotherapist? Gradually, we face up to the recognition, possible for anyone, of the human feelings with which this family are struggling. There are the feelings of bewilderment, guilt, the feelings of, 'Why have I been picked on?' and, of course, there are untouchable anxieties about the prognosis. Litigation cannot remove future problems.

These are feelings and anxieties that could very helpfully be ventilated between mother and physiotherapist and, thereby, it might be hoped that the work of physiotherapy could be disencumbered from this preoccupation with litigation. These are human problems rather than technical ones. Once again, it was mentioned that young physiotherapists, during their training, are warned away from giving patients technical explanations about their illnesses. They should leave this to the doctor. It is felt that this puts them in an impossible position but this may not be strictly true and there is this very clear feeling that the physiotherapist may use this as something to duck behind. There is no embargo on the recognition of anxiety, especially when it is interfering with the work of physiotherapy itself.

Incidentally, on this occasion Ms Yew became much more expansive than we have ever heard her before.

Case 79 (Ms Oak)

A lady of 73 with severe chronic rheumatoid arthritis was re-admitted as an emergency. She is an old patient of Ms Oak's, with severe disability. In the ambulance, on the way to hospital for routine treatment as an out-patient, the ambulance had to stop suddenly and she was pitched onto the floor, with her husband and the ambulance attendant on top of her. She has a spiral fracture of the femur and various other injuries. She is in quite a mess and told Ms Oak that she intends to sue the hospital.

Oddly, the cause of the accident was a patient walking out into the road from another hospital which the ambulance happened to be passing on the way.

This case appears to have been raised simply by association with Ms Yew's. The situation is less spooky than the previous case with its rare and extraordinary congenital affliction. There is more readiness to shoulder the moderate but real feelings of guilt, on behalf of the hospital, for a share of responsibility in the fresh injuries.

Ms Oak very firmly referred the patient to the doctor for medical advice and towards a solicitor for legal advice — although somewhat anxious lest we think she had been pushing the patient towards litigation. It seems to be more a question of clearing the air and clearing the field for the work of the physiotherapy they have to do together.

Forty-ninth meeting — Wednesday, 20th June, 1973

Case 80 (Ms Oak)

A depressing problem. A somewhat severe burnt-out rheumatoid arthritis, with a chronic empyema and an open drain from her right middle lobe. The whole picture is now severely aggravated by some rheumatoid arterial disease causing multiple ulcers at the extremities. These are very painful and do not respond to any treatment.

Ms Oak has been induced, rather against her better judgement, into giving ultraviolet therapy. She wanted to try it on an ulcer on one elbow first but was swiftly deflected from this, the doctor mentioning something about 'shining your magic lamps'. One gets a sense of a mixture of factors that have pushed Ms Oak and her colleagues off a determined professional approach to the condition, towards dabbling and magic. There is a mixture of pity and hostility towards this woman and I note that Ms Oak is able to say less about her, as a person, than she has ever said about any of her patients. We know that the woman is depressed, miserable, in a lot of pain, smokes a lot and has peroxide hair. She has been placed in a room of her own — again the same mixture of compassion and hostility.[1] Ms Oak appears to be regarded as some sort of expert on ulcers and is interested in them, certainly. She does sketch a picture of a more determined business-like approach as against her feeling that there has been a lot of dabbling, which has discredited a great many treatments, whether or not they need have been discredited. Meanwhile, the patient has suddenly started idealising Ms Oak and attaching the most inordinate hopes to the ultraviolet treatment, and, of course, Ms Oak is very worried about being in this false position.

Case 58 (Ms Sycamore) — follow-up

Her patient with the below-knee amputation. She got her final prosthesis and managed amazingly well with it, to Ms Sycamore's great satisfaction and surprise. Subsequently however, she developed a very tiny sore spot, which Ms Sycamore thought would be quite routine. She took her off the prosthesis and the pylon etc, expecting it to clear up, but in a couple of days it was worse. At the end of discussion the danger re-emerged (forgotten hitherto) that the amputation had not been high enough, since the original cellulitis, for which the amputation had been done, used to extend above the knee.

Meanwhile, most of the discussion was about the nature of Ms Sycamore's involvement and her sense, in retrospect, of having colluded inexplicably with this woman's very long stay in hospital — and the failure to use the time to best effect. In particular, she suddenly realised her own and the patient's blind-spot, in that the patient has never been on a bus or even thought of using public transport. This is side by side with the ostensible intention of resuming work as a schoolteacher in September. I link this with Ms Sycamore's experience of being swallowed up, unable to separate herself from the patient's experience of this amputation, because Ms Sycamore herself does not experience it as a routine. She has not handled one before and not seen a prosthesis, any more than the patient had. In spite of the usual emphasis on the need to really understand the patient's feelings and not to be lost in the medical world, here we see the dangers of the opposite process, where the therapist is lost in the patient's world and unable to maintain sufficient professional detachment, to be fully competent on the job.

Case 51 (Ms Sycamore) – follow-up
Her other follow-up was old Mr Dodds, the man (of 80 odd) with the shoulder who used to do Christian good works. He is now re-attending for something else and treated by somebody else. Ms Sycamore is keeping her distance in the face of greetings as a long lost friend.

Note
1 Single-bedded side-wards are liable to be reserved for privileged patients or for those who are regarded as too distressing to be tolerated in the main ward.

Fiftieth meeting – Wednesday, 4th July, 1973

Case 81 (Ms Poplar)
This is again the problem of an intrusion or a distraction. The girl presented is a young woman with PID (pelvic inflammatory disease), probably gonorrhoeal, and is allegedly the victim of a gang bang. The girl is excitable, endlessly demanding and has the whole staff running around in circles with her needs. At first she got Ms Poplar joining in, picking things up, fetching and carrying, but Ms Poplar soon stopped and tries to keep away. She is not really treating this girl in any direct way at all, but if she is treating somebody in the next bed the girl will appear under or around the curtain. The girl is obviously very disturbed and there does not really seem to be a genuine question of the physiotherapist having any real brief with her. It would only be a question of using the credentials of the physiotherapist to make an approach, if one were bent on so doing. The picture is rounded off by a further episode in which the girl was found with her feet dangling out of the first or second-floor window, then wanted to know what all the fuss was about – she was only cooling her feet on a hot day. As a result of this episode, all the windows are nailed down and can only open slightly at the top.

The case seemed mainly to represent the way in which the energies of professional staff may be wasted or uselessly expended on signals that turn them on and get them excited – Ms Poplar in particular – to the detriment of their work with other patients. (This is made concrete in the seminar by the way we, in turn, are in danger of being landed with this case, instead of having other more appropriate cases to discuss.)

However, the matter was enlarged by a discussion of Ms Poplar's dealings with the young woman in the next bed, who is a sociologist. She is also in for PID although history does not relate whether it is gonorrhoeal as well.

The point is that Ms Poplar found herself rather helpless in discussions with this young woman – overawed by her being a professional sociologist – although the conversation sounds somewhat futile, with much anger about the other patient having caused the nailing down of the windows. It was quite difficult to get the seminar to face the fact that the disturbance was very much around anxiety and the specific suicidal impulse displayed. The temptation was to collude with vague annoyance in general about loss of ventilation on a hot day.

All sorts of possible opportunities were missed, where this young woman might have been helped to express some of her feelings about her own condition; and even to touch on the possibilities of feeling depressed, suicidal impulses etc, instead of being able, in the event, to distance it all, right over the horizon, into the other girl, who can be viewed as a remote sort of underworld specimen. It is interesting to see Ms Poplar tempted into interfering in the case of the barmy girl (but resisting), and then shying off the sort of appropriate tentative work she might have been trying with the sociologist who was actually her patient. The seminar expressed some of the recurrent anxieties about stirring up more than you can deal with, fantasies of causing God knows what scene with the second patient, although they did see, once it was broached, that a tactful, realistic sort of conversation, admitting the discussion of anxieties, would not be likely to cause any breakdown that was not there already.

Case 82 (Ms Lime)

This was almost a non-case in that she appeared to have no problem at all with it and was simply reporting an aspect of work that you can only do in the domiciliary situation. This is an elderly lady who has had strokes, on and off, for about eight years and Ms Lime has treated her over this time. The recent strokes occurred after a long gap of several years. As well as traditional physiotherapy, Ms Lime is also and indeed mainly engaged in providing aspects of personal help which many physiotherapists would dispute as being inappropriate to their role. This includes assistance with dressing, bathing and so forth, and teaching the husband how to do these things too. She works with them mainly together and there are only brief moments when the husband is out of the room to make a cup of tea etc. The others questioned the effect of this perpetual chaperone on every conversation. There is also a daughter of the house who is grown-up and out at work all day. Somebody did wonder whether the husband must feel a bit hag-ridden with all these women around. The GP's wife, an ex-Bart's sister, also comes in to help, in a rather similar way. Ms Lime is going to drive them down to a special hotel for disabled people so that they can have a week or two's break shortly. It emerged from the conversation, quite clearly, that the break would be for the husband, who does all the cooking etc, and it obviously came as something of a surprise to the wife to see it that way – as if she had not quite realised how pinned down he is.

Fifty-first meeting – Wednesday, 18th July, 1973

The last session

Mainly follow-ups and discussion. The opening continued a spontaneous discussion about 'agency' colleagues, ie temporary staff employed from agencies rather than directly by the hospital. Members of the seminar appeared to be aware of some paranoid attitudes to these people. Colleagues tend to see them as lacking dedication and loyalty, resenting the fact that they are opting for higher pay and better hours — and, by association with other remarks, for better conditions. Ms Teak had mentioned some instance of casualty officers, who were supposed to be agency doctors, who had ditched the job because conditions were not good enough. She was inclined to be shocked at this dereliction of professional duty but the main trend was to gather a sense of something much more peculiar about the longstanding traditions of craven subservience, idealisation of superiors, and the putting up with bloody awful things that should not be put up with.[1]

In other words, we have to ask, 'dedication and loyalty to what?' I stated my further thought that some of this was about our ending today and unconscious residual feelings of resentment there. There was an element of mutual reproach involved and the sense that we were stopping because of disloyalty, lack of dedication etc by person or persons unknown.

Ms Elm is about to take up a job with a brewery — as an occupational physiotherapist. It is not clear whether she will be working under or with doctors, but the main impression is that she will be working very independently, as mistress of her own establishment of one person, herself. She will be paid something well above the top rate for teaching hospital physiotherapy. Although leading the discussion about disenchantment with physiotherapy and the wish to get out, she does also specify the particular frustrations she got into as a physiotherapy teacher. She felt particularly frustrated watching somebody else's hand on the patient and wanting to get her own hands in. I took this up as a reminder of one of our great gaps or blanks in the touching. The seminar has talked very much as if physiotherapy is a no-touch technique. There was general agreement that we had done this except for rare moments. Ms Elm reminded us that she has gone through (? is still in) a phase of revulsion from touching any patient, male or female. She does not think she is particularly no-touch person outside her work — she is probably about average, she thinks. Ms Lime surprisingly, confessed that she used to be (? still is) rather inclined to dislike too much contact and has had to get over this.

Case 58 (Ms Sycamore) — follow-up
The woman with the below-knee amputation. Discussion of Ms Poplar's case a couple of weeks ago suddenly made her realise that this case had been, for her, a red herring, a distraction. She now thinks that she (like the hospital team) has been far too preoccupied with this woman, who is really a psychiatric case, and that it would have been better to cut her losses. The goals for physiotherapy should have been more limited and the psychological problem acknowledged as such and directed towards more appropriate handling. This has led her to put the matter to one of the doctors to do something accordingly. This led on to the question of who to ask and, interestingly, she chose the new houseman. She reckons that the surgeon is himself far too deeply involved and, anyway, will never stop for two seconds to talk. The Registrar knows all about it, but has gone to the other extreme and is lodged in obstinate total disinterest. So her hopes are placed with the new houseman who does not know anything about it but may, at least, be open-minded and free to act.

Case 82 (Ms Lime) – follow-up

The lady with the stroke. Good progress has been made and she is now able to dress herself, using her good hand. Ms Lime's use of relaxation techniques to achieve voluntary relaxation of the spastic arm led to some impassioned discussion. Ms Elm's physiological knowledge was affronted and she wanted to insist that you cannot voluntarily relax a spastic arm. Yet Ms Lime has been doing just that with the patient! Behind this lie questions as to which god you worship – Ms Elm struggles to disencumber herself from worship of medical gods, physiological science etc. Ms Lime is suspected of worshiping relaxation techniques as a universal panacea. Ms Poplar points out that 'she seems to want to treat everything with relaxation'. Ms Poplar herself thinks that natural childbirth is 'a load of cobblers'.

And there we had to leave it.

Note
1 This was also discussed from another angle. Some of this traditional martyred behaviour may be designed as a protection against the resentment, by ill patients, of healthy staff. If one is overworked and badly treated, it is much harder for patients to express their complaints and their envy.

Retrospect

Eventually the group reconvened to discuss a draft of this report. We all agreed that we were looking back on something that had stopped in mid-flight rather than a completed process. Some lessons are fairly clear and certain whilst large areas of physiotherapy are still totally unexplored by us.

We have learnt how physiotherapy is 'a remedial profession', inspired with the goals of function and cure whereas, in reality, physiotherapists carry the most disabled and incurable people. The realistic aims will often be the achievement of quite marginal improvement in function for a temporary period and, sometimes, nothing more than the hope of lifting morale in patients and doctors.

The tradition of medical primacy, together with the fact that most doctors are men and most physiotherapists are women, combine to create certain configurations that occupied much of our time – and which have been discussed in the previous sections.

The seminar itself was subject to the influence of certain features that moulded our work. The time restriction, our limited life-span together, was an overriding factor and I doubt whether we could have covered much more ground than we did, whoever we had managed to enlist. However, we were very conscious of the many areas of physiotherapy that were not covered in our work. We should have welcomed the viewpoint of colleagues from these fields even though we could not, in the time, have done justice to a much wider clinical panorama. We were aware of some of our restrictions – and were probably blind to others. Work with children and work with the mentally handicapped would probably merit a seminar of its own. Work in residential institutions for the disabled, other than hospitals, is also a field almost on its own – as is the field of rehabilitation, in which physiotherapy enters as one component in an educational and developmental programme. We did not deal with ante-natal training to any depth (although one member of the seminar is an expert in this field), nor (except for one case) with relaxation techniques. We discussed massage mainly in the abstract, rather than in relation to specific cases; and we did not hear about manipulation (except for examination and manipulation under anaesthesia, by surgeons, which came in quite often). We had no male physiotherapists and no blind physiotherapists — two classes within the profession who must encounter some different problems from this group.

However, we have made a start.

Index of cases

Ms Ash's cases (3)

Case no 6: woman with sciatica: an ex-physiotherapist
First reported on 15th March, 1972. Referred 'to get her moving somehow'. Ms Ash suspects physical lesion, notices temperature difference between the legs - but cannot act to take it any further. The woman is not really in the role of patient and not really in the role of colleague.

Follow-up 22nd March, 1972. First follow-up mainly for Ms Ash to register hurt sense of being misunderstood by the seminar.

Follow-up 22nd June, 1972. This came up in the context of a discussion about colleagues as patients. No real change has occurred in this case and the struggle continues. Ms Oak inherited this patient and further follow-ups are reported with her cases nine months later.

Case no 7: woman of 38: mastectomy for cancer of breast
Reported 22nd March, 1972. She is attending for radiotherapy and physiotherapy. The ostensible problem is an unexplained quarrel between the patient and a previous physiotherapist, resulting in her transfer to Ms Ash by the department head.
  The real problem is that the physiotherapist does not know what the patient is supposed to know about the diagnosis. Policy seems to be that it is 'better not to know', either about the cancer or about the previous row. How well does this work?
  Many preoccupations of this case are linked with matters of surface appearance, the attractiveness of the patient, the perfection of the scar, as against the distress of encountering mutilation, or seeing other disabled patients and ugly sights in the physiotherapy department.
  These physiotherapists also suspect that surgeons are irrationally fearful of physiotherapy following cancer operations.

Case no 15: the blind physiotherapist: a colleague
Reported 22nd June, 1972. The patients think she is marvellous but her

188

colleagues find her pushing and inconsiderate. She wants to push her patients in first all the time and nobody likes to make her take her turn. Similarly she escapes the chores of clearing up, although quite capable of doing her share. When finally clear that this was a problem of personality and not one of blindness, Ms Ash felt able to tick her off and gain a considerable improvement.

But what about other forms of blindness in colleagues? And, are we, unawares, equally resentful of all those patients whose disabilities give us work?

Ms Beech's cases (2)

She was in the preliminary series of five seminars and re-joined for a couple of months, a year later.

Case no 5: young man from Syria, having traction for neck pains

Reported 15th March, 1972. The treatment caused intense panic at first but this was overcome and good progress achieved. We discussed the use, problems and management of frightening treatments. Subsequently, there is study of trick-movements to diagnose the residual psychological component. The treatment is stuck.

How much of all this is really about misgivings concerning private practice, misgivings about charlatanry, and doubts about frightening treatments. Is a private fee simply the rate for the job or is it something illicit, signifying guilt for the paid therapist and important overtones of punishment for the patient?

Case no 62: woman in her 60s: facial palsy.

First reported 28th February, 1973. The patient is referred for daily electrical treatment and the physiotherapists think this nonsensical. Allegedly, the doctor promised the patient a complete recovery (the prognosis is really uncertain) and Ms Beech is humiliated and enraged. Incidentally, she learns that the patient is struggling with a daughter in mental hospital.

The first discussion centred upon the collusion of the physiotherapists (all women) to maintain the doctor as an unseen idiot or bogeyman whereas it should be quite possible to go and see him to establish some sensible dialogue.

Follow-up 14th March, 1973. Ms Beech has been unable to reach the doctor owing to a barrier of secretaries, nurses and her own superintendent. She confronted the latter politely but firmly whereupon a tremendous public row ensued. However, it has resulted in an arrangement for regular meetings between the physical medicine consultant and the different physiotherapists; and he has now discussed the prognosis with the patient in a more balanced way.

Follow-up 28th March, 1973. Ms Beech finally meets the consultant. He is a charming, open-minded young man, nothing like the fantasy that had been built-up. We are left wondering what part such fantasy-objects play in the organisation of a predominantly women's profession. The temptation to idealise physical treatments and ingenious mechanical gadgets is, at depth, linked with the same ambivalent need to idealise exaggeratedly masculine authority figures.

Meanwhile, the doctor is left unaware of the situation surrounding him. Ms Beech left the seminar at this point.

Ms Elder's case

Case no 8: lady in her 70s: arthritis — breast cancer as incidental finding.
Reported 22nd March, 1972. She is in hospital for a tibial osteotomy for advanced rheumatoid arthritis and osteo-arthritis and the house surgeon finds a lump in the breast. The patient is old, rather deaf and not very bright Who should tell her that the lump must be removed? And how is this to be done since she is deaf, dull and afraid and nobody dares to use the word 'cancer'?

The surgical team appears to be a happy interdisciplinary group but it is not clear who is best fitted to inform the patient and obtain her consent. Is this really a job for the social worker (to whom it is delegated) who may be best at talking but knows least about the surgical treatment? What is the role of the physiotherapist in such a situation?

Ms Elder was in the initial trial run of seminars but could not attend the main series. This was the only case of hers that we discussed.

Ms Elm's cases (10)

Case no 4: middle-aged man: osteo-arthritis of hips — arthroplasties
First reported 8th March, 1972. He has had several unsuccessful operations and is about to have another. He seems addicted to surgery. Ms Elm disagrees with all this and incurs his emnity by discussing his possible discharge. She thinks he plays off the surgeon behind her back and also exploits the rivalry that may exist between Ms Elm and her attractive students.

Follow-up 6th September, 1972. She ran across him in the outpatient clinic and, although aware of previous coolness, was shocked to be roundly abused. He has now had a fifth arthroplasty (three on one hip, two on the other)!

Case no 9: man aged 52: Colles's fracture
Reported on 28th March, 1972. A tremulous terrified man, looking nearer 70 than 52, who is not recovering from a broken wrist. It occurred when he was drunk and his only pleasure in life appears to be the pub. His melancholy and isolation are evident in the story but not properly faced. Instead, the physiotherapist identifies herself with him unconsciously. She seems to feel equally isolated as if she too has to carry everything by herself. She seems to have no perception of a GP in the background and, if at all, only vague remote colleagues on another planet.

Case no 14: man aged 48: rheumatoid arthritis
Reported 8th June, 1972. This was a case of sudden and severe onset, carrying a poor prognosis. This is important since the patient works as a docker and his main interest is as a wrestling trainer.

He is not really sent to the Physiotherapy Department to 'have treatment': the physical medicine consultant, who referred the patient, has specifically charged Ms Elm with the task of helping him to grasp the situation. She is quite unable to succeed in getting him to change his expectations of complete swift recovery. This impedes treatment.

This is another case in which Ms Elm and the patient both seem very isolated (see case 9).

Case no 18: porter: neck pain
First reported 6th July, 1972. This followed a minor accident at work, with no perceptible injury. However, he gets all sorts of physical treatment and nobody will face the diagnosis which they all know — that there is no physical condition to treat. There is some thought about 'compensation neurosis' but the real fear is to be involved in his wish to discuss himself and his marriage — and there is good evidence that he does want to confide.

The physiotherapists wonder if he 'needs a floozie' and slowly realise that they may be occupying just such a role when they provide quack remedies and physical gratifications whilst deceiving themselves about the indications.

Follow-up 20th July, 1972. A couple of weeks later it is reported that he has disappeared from treatment. Should Ms Elm write to him, phone the GP or what?

Case no 24: middle-aged man: cervical spondylosis
Reported 27th July, 1972. The diagnosis is very uncertain and the doctor's prescribed treatment is 'try traction'. The physiotherapists are enraged and bewildered by the patient's peculiarly obscure way of talking and the intrusiveness of his behaviour.

Possibly, on his side, he is made worse by the obscurantist handling of his case, where a more open discussion of the uncertainty could be more calming than a bustling face of efficient activity.

Case no 31: postman with bachache
Reported 27th September, 1972. He is a pathetic, weedy little man who fell on his bottom a few months ago. Severe backache returns whenever physiotherapy stops.

Ms Elm is astonished at the hostility her report generates in a very nice surgical Registrar but she was not able to discuss this further with him (the Registrar).

Case no 33: woman with backache
Reported 11th October, 1972. The case (so far as the seminar is concerned)

191

centres around a curious rivalry-cum-co-operation between the surgical registrar and the physiotherapist. She notices the weird gait which he can then demonstrate to be hysterical – but then perversely treats by suggesting a month in bed at home. The evident matrimonial problem is ignored – or indeed aggravated – by this course.

Behind the aggrieved feeling of being 'only the physiotherapist' there is secret triumph over such doctors who act stupidly whereas they might sometimes really be quite ready to learn from the physiotherapist.

Case no 34: old lady: generalised osteo-arthritis
Reported 11th October, 1972. Another instance of the disliked chronic patient, attending long after the time when any good is being done by the treatment. The physiotherapist is so preoccupied with her knowledge that the patient and the doctor are making a fool of her that she cannot act constructively. These problems of status and scorn poison any legitimate use of placebo treatments and interfere with reasonable discussion of alternative arrangements.

Case 39: man aged 25: osteosarcoma of tibia – amputation and death
Reported 15th November, 1972. His mother could not bear to see him until he had a prosthesis for the empty trouser leg. The waves of disturbing feelings about this case include changing identifications with the patient, mother, father and wife. There are special anxieties about the nature of maternal love and a sense that it may have unattractive narcissistic components. There may be a guilty feeling of relief, when death removes something which has become ugly.

Case 44: woman aged 75: Parkinsonism
First reported 29th November, 1972. This is a private patient and Ms Elm is constantly pushed out of her professional role in a way that would never happen in her hospital work. There is enthusiastic progress at first but Ms Elm is soon caught up in rivalries amongst the grown-up children. Moreover, enthusiastic progress by-passes the more difficult problem of being 'with them' in their underlying fears. Even the diagnosis has to be veiled as 'features of Parkinsonism'. How might the family be involved in the treatment? What diagnostic skills and special techniques are necessary for domiciliary work?

Follow-up 13th December, 1972. It is reported that Ms Elm is struggling to ventilate the taboo subject of ageing in this family.

Follow-up 20th December, 1972. Things are turning very sour as Ms Elm is about to take a Christmas holiday. Moreover, although supposedly trying to get the patient to examine problems and anxieties about ageing and the future, it emerges that Ms Elm herself seems brightly to have been hoping to bow out of the case, after a short period of treatment.

Follow-up 10th January, 1973. Ms Elm is now awkwardly embroiled with the family and wishing she could get out. Inexperience of private work makes her feel awkward about fees and susceptible to all sorts of invasive behaviour from various members of the family. Moreover, unorthodox methods, which may be so useful in domiciliary work, require a degree of automatic sure-footedness that may be undermined by constant discussion in the seminar. Ms Elm has, supposedly become indispensible to this patient and her family but they succeed in treating her however they like.

Ms Hazel's case

Case no 1: girl aged 15 with backache

Reported 1st March, 1972. She is unable to go to school. Treatment drags on for a year to little avail. The medical referral for traction was wrong since there was excessive mobility already. There are also many psychological problems about the case. Ms Hazel sees no way of initiating better treatment and no way of communicating her diagnostic impressions (physical or psychological) to her medical colleagues.

There are at least two obstacles to effective work in this case. On the one hand there is the impulse to keep things pleasant and the belief that it is always necessary for the patient to respect or like you. On the other hand there is the need to maintain appearances of respect over an undercurrent of contempt for 'superiors' — which presumably includes doctors.

The physiotherapist is thus in no position to help an adolescent girl who is herself torn between rebellion and concern for her adoptive parents — mother suspiciously nice and elegant, father with a recent coronary thrombosis.

Ms Hazel was in the initial trial run of seminars but could not attend the main series. This was the only case of hers that we discussed.

Ms Lime's cases (4)

Case no 48: baby 10 months old: spastic

First reported 20th December, 1972. The case centres around the professional isolation of the physiotherapist and the social isolation of the mother. The physiotherapist has never treated a spastic baby before, has to pick up the technique as best she can and wants advice from the seminar. Father is separated, mother is only about 20 and there is another three-year-old running about. They live with grandma.

Our difficulty in the seminar is to dislodge the physiotherapist from unspecified but pressing models of psychiatric social work based on multiple interviewing, history-taking and so forth. The seminar's aim is to clarify what might be the appropriate aspirations within the particular opportunities of work as a physiotherapist. Thus, it might be possible to engage the grandmother and the absent father in some of the necessary activities with the baby and thereby establish a working sense of whatever is possible within this family.

Follow-ups on 10th January, 1973, 17th January, 1973, 24th January, 1973 and 31st January, 1973. It remains difficult for the seminar to get past the social preoccupations towards a realistic sense of Ms Lime's actual work with the mother and baby. There are broken appointments, the husband never turns up and it emerges finally that he is under arrest for robbery with violence.

Case no 64: ante-natal classes
First reported 14th March, 1973. There appears to be a pleasant working co-operation with the physiotherapist in the labour ward in contrast with much mutual suspicion and resentment in the ante-natal and post-natal situations. There, she feels isolated by the nurses and caught up in a style of work inimical to the communication of human feelings and anxieties.

Apart from a general expectation that the ante-natal classes should teach exercises and physical procedures but not encourage talk, there is a specific embargo on physiotherapists 'answering any questions'. Apparently, a physiotherapist once nearly caused the death of a woman by her failure to appreciate the significance of an incipient antepartum haemorrhage.

Follow-up 30th May, 1973. It seems she is unable to start ante-natal training classes at the hospital owing to opposition by the midwives. However, there is the possibility of a research project in co-operation with the gynaecologist and X University.

Case no 73: woman in post-natal ward: episiotomy
Reported 15th May, 1973. The patient had been told, correctly, by the gynaecologist that her sutures were absorbable and would not need to be removed. However, the pieces of suture remaining on the surface do often have to be removed and the patient complains to Ms Lime.

This was a particular example in a more general discussion about the problem of patients who feel that promises and explanations have been dishonest, and who feel betrayed.

Case no 82: old lady: multiple strokes
First reported 4th July, 1973. This is a domiciliary case showing possibilities of an unconventional and flexible approach that is more appropriate in the patient's home than in the hospital gymnasium. Ms Lime uses her knowledge of physiotherapy techniques to teach the patient and her husband how to manage better around the house, consolidating the importance of whatever the patient should be able to do for herself and teaching the husband how to be most effective in helping her over the more tricky difficulties — for example, in getting dressed.

Some of Ms Lime's procedures range between social work and ordinary 'good neighbourliness', and the GP's wife also helps out. Other members of the seminar wonder if there are not too many women on top of this poor husband.

Follow-up 18th July, 1973. The application of relaxation techniques to reduce spasticity — probably a spill-over from Ms Lime's ante-natal work. The seminar are anxious that this all sounds rather unscientific but Ms Lime 'believes in it' and it seems to work. The physiotherapists' lack of faith in many of the techniques they have to employ has been a recurrent anxiety emerging throughout the seminar.

Ms Mahogany's cases (9)

Case no 16: a young man in hospital with miliary tuberculosis
First reported 29th June, 1972. The problem is the hostility of staff and other patients alike towards this patient who is always moaning and miserable. He is a West Indian and suspected of being homosexual, but some of the primitive feeling he generates may be due to the prolonged uncertainty and obscurity of his diagnosis and everybody's unadmitted fear of catching something.

Follow-up 6th July, 1972. He became more ill. Everyone became more sympathetic and he, in turn, is more co-operative. The chicken or the egg?

Case no 21: woman aged 23: removal of patella
Reported 20th July, 1972. Severe rehabilitation problems, and all sorts of techniques and tricks are to no avail.

The patient is immensely chatty and friendly but may, at depth, really be suspicious and resentful about the operation. It feels like a trick played on her while she was asleep and the difficulty is to help her to feel supported rather than tricked now. The recent death of mother is a further important factor in the case.

Case no 28: woman of 35: rheumatoid arthritis
Reported 20th September, 1972. A severe chronic case and Ms Mahogany wants to try out a new treatment. Slowly, she has to face the discovery that the patient is quite unco-operative and, at depth, totally opposed to mobilisation and recovery. She was previously treated at another hospital much nearer home. Her move to Ms Mahogany's hospital may have more to do with a flight from anxieties and pressures at home than with the ostensible fresh impetus for treatment. Thus, attempts to get her to chat about home life are swimming against the tide.

Case no 20
This patient is listed with Ms Poplar's cases.

Case no 30: middle-aged man: ulnar nerve injury
Reported 27th September, 1972. The case is a few months old and originally treated at another hospital. Ms Mahogany is caught between her junior, who does the treatment and her senior colleague, who has a special interest in cases of this type.

Moreover, the condition has been badly neglected. Ms Mahogany's senior suspects self-inflicted injury and now urges intensive daily treatment, which may be unrealistic. Ms Mahogany sympathises with the patient, who fears that he could lose his job (civil servant), in the process.

We see the need for much carefully collected information, whereas there is a sort of taboo against physiotherapists taking any responsibility for a systematic enquiry. Their ethos is to 'pick up' whatever you can, with nobody noticing, as you go along.

Case no 35: woman aged 56: Colles's fracture
First reported 18th October, 1972. She is on the Disabled Persons Register, although apparently able-bodied. The physiotherapist has difficulty in getting out of an accusatory role and into an investigating/diagnostic one. This is a recurrent result of the physiotherapist feeling she has no licence to take the patient into a room and get the history, instead of slyly 'slipping in' questions between exercises.

Follow-up 1st November, 1972. It turns out that the woman was not actually on the Disabled Persons Register but was trying to get on to it. The physiotherapists are very angry with patients they perceive as greedy and with doctors and social workers who collude: and this anger disturbs work. Meanwhile, the patient has broken off treatment.

Case no 45: man aged about 50: severe rheumatoid arthritis
First reported 6th December, 1972. After three years' treatment he is severely disabled and the condition is static. The presenting problem now is to get him off treatment and out of the department. The physiotherapists feel unable to make the doctors shoulder their own problems — just like the patient himself. Feelings run high but something always goes wrong when they try to discharge him.
   He weighs 16 stone. Do the staff resent him because he is a greedy, lazy, exploiting man or is there rather a collusion to keep him like a helpless fat baby? Are the staff too disturbed by their own anxieties at the sight of a healthy man stricken and crippled in his prime? The psychological facts are hard to face, eg his grandchild, with spina bifida, had to have both feet amputated.

Follow-up 13th December, 1972. He is taken on a 'home visit' but the escort is told not to bring him back! Meanwhile, the seminar discover how unexpectedly angry they are at the thought of having to wipe his bottom for him — even though this is not at all likely to arise in reality.

Case no 50: woman in her 50s: ruptured Achilles tendon
First reported 10th January, 1973. This is a rather forbidding, superior university reader. She made no progress and walked so atrociously that Ms Mahogany became angry enough to tick her off and, thereby, precipitate a nasty row in public. (Very unlike Ms Mahogany.)
   This simmers down but the patient now claims treatment for her knees ('I have a psychosomatic disorder of the knee . . . ') and also believes she has gout — which she has not.
   The case throws up a discussion of the way patients may feel unnecessarily humiliated by treatment routines, like putting them into hospital shorts. Could Ms Mahogany steer this patient towards the psychotherapy she appears to need? And should we recognise that some patients are not suitable for physiotherapy?

Follow-up 7th February, 1973. Things have improved since the row. This might be in spite of the row or because of it but is probably a success belonging to the general practitioner, who knows how to manage her.

Ms Oak's cases (15)

Case no 2: middle-aged woman: weak, painful foot following minor injury
Reported 1st March, 1972. Severe disability had persisted in spite of every
out-patient treatment, following a minor injury three years ago. Finally,
the physical medicine consultant admits the patient, expressly for Ms Oak
to cure by hook or by crook.

The seminar are enraged, feeling that physiotherapists are always being
humiliated and exploited — but they seem even more upset by the complete
success of this management, within three weeks. Does the doctor know
what the physiotherapist can do better than she herself knows? Does *his*
blessing and prestige enable *her* to do what he cannot do? And how was it
done?

Case no 11: Spanish-Gibraltarian woman of 48: bedridden with disseminated
sclerosis
First reported 25th May, 1972. She has been an in-patient for 3½ years. The
nursing staff and house physicians come and go, the consultant visits weekly
but Ms Oak is the one person who has been most closely and continuously
involved with the care of this patient. She has become, in some ways, a
substitute mother and this involves the pair of them in an unexpected range
of conflicting feelings. Sometimes Ms Oak wants to see the patient taken out
for a walk in the sun . . . but at other times she wishes the agony were over
and the bed empty.

Foreign herself, she is liable to become entangled in the patient's varying
feelings about the English, Gibraltarians, and other foreigners. Part of Ms
Oak's job seems occasionally to be spent in occupying the role of cruel mother
or some other villain. This can enable other staff to be idealised (by contrast)
— which is sometimes an advantage, although painful to Ms Oak.

Follow-ups 15th June, 1972, 22nd June, 1972, 18th October, 1972 and
1st November, 1972. The case struggles on with bursts of feeling — variously
angry or erotic. There was a strange flurry reported in October, when the
staff nurse was getting married and the patient amazed Ms Oak by proposing that they go away and make a baby together. Hints of past psychotic
breakdown emerge.

Case no 14: woman with disseminated sclerosis
Reported 22nd June, 1972. The woman infuriates Ms Oak by walking 'for
the consultant' on his weekly round, but not for her in the gym. She narrow-
ly avoids losing her temper and realises, suddenly, that the patient has method
in it. She confronts the patient with her understanding that this behaviour
is designed to ensure that Ms Oak persists in working hard with her and that
the consultant is gratified by the results and will give his blessing to a pro-
longation of treatment. Ms Oak helps the patient realise that it may be
better to make progress than to prolong the treatment and remain in a chair
— and she is rewarded by rapid improvement.

Case no 23: lady aged 81: broken leg and conjunctivitis
First reported 27th July, 1972. The consultant decides that the patient can
be discharged, on his weekly ward round. Somehow the physiotherapist is
landed with the job of arranging it. The patient is in tears and Ms Oak is
somewhat lost in the role of mothering people.

Follow-up 6th September, 1972. The seminar has helped Ms Oak to dis-
entangle herself from an inappropriate task. It then emerges that the entire
staff group had deluded themselves into seeing this lady as a member of a
united loving family, with a false mystery as to why she would not go home.
   Actually, a meeting with the family left the medical social worker in
tears and Ms Oak providing cups of tea. However, a successful trial visit
home was followed by discharge a few days later.

Case no 27: an old lady: another discharge problem
First reported 13th September, 1972. A surprising and unprecedented row
with the ward sister over arrangements to be made and sharing the burden.
Strong feelings are exposed by ill-timed discussions on an empty stomach
and in the context of excitement and envy associated with the new out-
patient unit which is about to open.

Follow-up 27th September, 1972. Now it has all blown over.

Case no 32: woman with rheumatoid arthritis
Reported 27th September, 1972. The patient is kept in the gym and late
back for lunch. Is this a facet of normal concern or is it connected with
some curious excessive concern?

Case no 36: a middle-aged man with an inoperable cerebral tumour
First reported 8th October, 1972. The usual conspiracy of silence and
nobody knows what to say to anybody else. Meanwhile, the patient's
wife has to go into a mental hospital for a weekend.

Follow-up 8th November, 1972. The hospital management structure allows
the experience and responsibility to be fragmented amongst different people
in different wards and units. The physiotherapists may sometimes carry
most of the continuity — and anguish. Moreover, they are the most
obviously 'fit' people around the hospital and therefore more subject to
envy by patients — and even by colleagues.

Follow-up 22nd November, 1972. A nice letter from patient's wife to say
that he died peacefully at home and thanking everybody for the care shown.

Case no 43: a woman: post-cholecystectomy and chronic bronchitis
Reported 29th November, 1972. She spoke sharply to a woman about
smoking whereupon the woman disclosed that she recognised her (Ms Oak)
as having treated her child four years ago. The child — as well as three
others — died of spina bifida: so she had something to smoke about.

Did Ms Oak really, at depth, recognise the woman?

Case no 57: woman aged 39: mobilisation after laminectomy
First reported 24th January, 1973. The problem is to get the woman walking.
Her histrionic antics infuriate Ms Oak. (The operation is for a prolapsed
intervertebral disc with neurological physical signs.)

Follow-up 7th February, 1973. She wants a psychiatrist called in but the
neuro-surgeon predicts, correctly, that this will all settle if they can get her
walking somehow. Is the physiotherapist somehow picking up some of
the patient's primitive fury against the surgeon who inflicts operations? She
finds it very hard to tell the surgeon that she cannot treat this patient: but
then it cools, whereupon the ward nursing staff succeed in a few days and
the woman is walking normally.

Follow-up 14th February, 1973. There appear to be themes about interdisciplinary rivalries and about nasty foreigners. Nurses can sometimes
perform 'physiotherapy' more successfully than the physiotherapists.

Case no 61: middle-aged man with cerebral tumour
Reported 28th February, 1973. The tumour is inoperable and the prognosis
is bad. However, the physiotherapist is vague in her own mind and the
patient meets the usual conspiracy of silence. This leads to difficulties in
physiotherapy and a failure to grasp possible priorities in his management.

Follow-up 11th May, 1973. Patient has now died at home.

Case no 6: woman with sciatica: an ex-physiotherapist
*First reported by Ms Ash 15th March, 1972. First reported by Ms Oak
21st March, 1973 (see Ms Ash's cases).* Ms Oak has inherited the case from
Ms Ash and the position seems to be exactly as it was. We still have the
feeling that maybe she should be re-investigated although she has already
been through the departments of two teaching hospitals.

Follow-up 11th April, 1973. Ms Oak discovers that there is a young daughter
with asthma but does not really establish any convincing rapport with this
patient. Should she be removed from doctors and physical treatments for
psychological investigation? Nobody can decide the diagnosis.

Follow-up 9th May, 1973. Some change but hardly an improvement.
Weight-reduction and therapy to improve posture has produced a new pain
in the shoulder.

*Case no 67: middle-aged woman: stiff neck, admitted for manipulation
under anaesthetic (MUA)*
Reported 28th March, 1973. The condition is believed to be hysterical.
Previous MUAs made no difference and showed normal mobility. Ms Oak
finds herself, unwittingly, gathering the psychological information which
begins to make the symptoms intelligible. There is a suicidal son and a

199

husband who nearly strangled her. A psychiatric referral can now be made, with this extra information.

Case no 70: gym teacher aged about 38: hysteria
First reported 9th May, 1973. On admission she is diagnosed and treated as severe acute rheumatoid arthritis. After 10 days this is recognised as hysteria and the patient is transferred to the psychiatric ward. In contrast to most cases of this type, the patient remains popular and there is none of the usual rancour.

Follow-up 30th May, 1973. Ms Oak still visits the patient in the psychiatric ward. A course of psychotherapy is planned.

Case no 79: lady aged 73: rheumatoid arthritis and road accident; litigation
Reported 13th June, 1973. An old patient is involved in an accident in the ambulance on the way for routine treatment. She is felt to have a good case for sueing the hospital but, once this is faced, nobody seems very unhappy about it.

Case no 80: woman with severe burnt-out rheumatoid arthritis and chronic empyema
Reported 20th June, 1973. There are painful intractable ulcers at the extremities and the physiotherapist, against her better judgement, is induced to 'shine your magic lamps . . . ' (ultra-violet irradiation). Treatment has degenerated into futile dabbling. Treatments keep changing and become discredited − perhaps unnecessarily.

Ms Poplar's cases (11)

Case no 13: Italian ex-athletics star aged 32: traumatic paraplegia
First reported 15th June, 1972.
Follow-ups 29th June, 1972; 6th July, 1972; 13th July, 1972; 20th July, 1972; 6th September, 1972; and 25th October, 1972. The problem is his failure to make any progress and the outbursts of screaming and other (sometimes violent) disturbance whenever he is pressed. Otherwise, he is a handsome, chatty and attractive man and there is much display of friendly banter between times. The hospital is due to close down shortly and he is awaiting a vacancy to go to Stoke Mandeville − special unit for treatment of paraplegics.
  During the subsequent follow-ups there is a tale of struggle but no real progress. There is a sense of two volatile people colliding repeatedly. However, although there are hints of brief minor improvement when Ms Poplar is on holiday or when the house physician institutes some other treatment, he has been discharged from a number of other hospitals before owing to the disturbance he creates and his failure to make much progress.

Case no 20: gorgeous Gussie, aged 58: osteo-arthritis of knees and post-encephalitic Parkinsonism
First reported 13th July, 1972. 'An old woman of 58' has been attending three times a week for 20 or 30 years and seems to be a weirdly picturesque, antique patient, attached to an 'elderly' (also in his 50s!) consultant who is gentle and courtly — both being relics of a byegone age, in Ms Poplar's eyes. *The hospital is closing down shortly.* The antiquarian ethos collides with the physiotherapist's commitment to youth and recovery.

Follow-up 20th September, 1972. The patient has been transferred to Ms Mahogany's hospital, to an astonishingly different regime. She has had a tibial osteotomy and, with more energetic management, looks younger and even 'quite attractive'. However, they still agree that she is 'quite mad'. Her Dopa (for the Parkinsonism) was reduced during surgery and she writes, 'Dear Sir or Madam' to Ms Poplar, asking her to intervene to get the dose restored.

Case no 25: Andy Capp type with cervical spondylosis
Reported 27th July, 1972. Collar will not fit. She has tried everything including a referral elsewhere but somehow there is an agreement between courtly consultant and another of his antique patients that Ms Poplar cannot fit a collar. The impression is of two men agreeing that a girl cannot do something practical. Somehow, a few of these problem patients may channel off ill-feeling leaving a general sense that otherwise Ms Poplar and the consultant get on famously.

Case no 26: woman with disseminated sclerosis
Reported 6th September, 1972. There are problems due to the impending closure of the hospital. No sensible arrangements are being made for this patient's future treatment owing to the pressure to sustain the same mystery about the future of the hospital as there is about the patient's medical prognosis. A bewildering and uncomfortable atmosphere is created. Beneath the surface there is provocation and inappropriate excitement, covered by a thin layer of 'reassurance' and a charade of 'management' of the problem. Anxiety cannot be squarely faced.

Case no 42: no specific patient, general problems of new job
Reported 22nd November, 1972. Problems of starting new job in a gynaeco-logical unit. She is the second physiotherapist there but has the impression that there is hardly enough work for one. The time is filled out by apparently futile rituals, silly regimes of exercises that nobody needs — for example, a post-operative regime of foot and ankle exercises following trivial opera-tions. However, she can see that there is a tremendous amount of psycho-logical disturbance around these gynaecological problems and a suspicion that some disturbed patients may be accessible via a routine with the physiotherapist although they would not countenance any approach from a social worker or psychiatrist. The physiotherapist has some role as therapeutic listener, if not counsellor, but the problem is to avoid losing sight of herself as a physiotherapist and turning into a gossip.

Case no 47: pregnant woman on bed rest for habitual abortion

First reported 13th December, 1972. A chatty attitude enables unusual confidences to be voiced by patients but undermines a professional demeanour suitable for handling them. Now — and worse — Ms Poplar receives even more awkward confidences concerning the patient's marriage from the house surgeon at a party. She is hamstrung with this unmentionable information.

Case no 59: Trinidad 'girl' of 30 having short-wave diathermy for sterility

Reported 14th February, 1973. This case goes with Ms Poplar's other case presented the same day — Case 60. She had a baby when she was about 14 and gave it up for adoption. Since then, she has never been able to become pregnant. She blurts out her depression to the physiotherapist who immediately ships her off to the social worker. Behind dicta about the right or wrong thing to do are the more specific issues about how Ms Poplar sees herself, her colleagues and her patients, eg seeing the 40-year-old social worker as an old, motherly, or even grandmotherly lady; and seeing the patient aged 30 as a girl. The case combines anxiety about ageing and about sterility.

Case no 60: woman with pulmonary valvotomy and 'threatened abortion', actually not pregnant

Reported 14th February, 1973. This case goes with Ms Poplar's other case presented the same day (Case no 59). This is again about sterility, ageing and strange reactions churned up in physiotherapist.

Case no 63: salpingectomy and sacroiliac strain

First reported 7th March, 1973. The patient is introduced as 'a typical middle-aged layabout' but, on discussion, her age turns out to be 42. Ms Poplar feels 30 years younger than this woman. The patient regales Ms Poplar with details of a bizarre and hectic sexual life, arousing all sorts of mixed feelings. There appear to be anxieties about 'middle-age' as a horrible decay of the sexual organs: and unconscious theories of 'therapy' are linked with compulsive sexual activity. The physiotherapist feels the threat of sexual feelings breaking out if she relaxes her normal defences and routines. However, the problem is not only one of sexual excitement but also involves anxieties about age and decay.

Follow-up 11th April, 1973. The previous discussion enabled Ms Poplar to see the patient in a more realistic perspective as neither an adolescent delinquent nor a senile and decrepit woman. On this basis she is able to tackle her more realistically, albeit very firmly and sharply. This may have got her on to her feet, for she promptly found a job and returned once more to thank Ms Poplar. Discussion of this case brought out important issues about feelings aroused in the therapist and some surprise about her capacity to affect the way a patient feels about herself.

The case also involved important issues about reality and danger as proper criteria for prohibitions (eg against lighting a fire in the wastepaper basket — as this woman did in her hostel bedroom one evening), instead of depending on arbitrary private moralities and rules.

Case no 66: a woman collapses and dies in an underground railway station
Reported 28th March, 1973. The physiotherapist, caught outside hospital
without her white coat on, is astonished at her own vulnerability. She is
terribly upset by the incident. Discussion exposes the envy of people like
surgeons who are pictured as doing clearly defined work with (allegedly)
well-established results. Physiotherapists − like psychotherapists − work
in a realm of vagueness and faith, for much of the time.

Case no 81: teenage girl with pelvic inflammatory disease (gonorrhoea)
Reported 4th July, 1973. Teenage girl, allegedly the victim of a 'gang-bang',
causes a commotion in the ward and engages Ms Poplar's concern. This
illustrates the problem of patients (and themes) who generate excitability
and anxiety in professional staff, distracting appropriate attention from
more appropriate work. The seminar discovered belatedly that our time
might have been better spent on a more 'normal' case. An episode in
which the patient dangled her legs out of a third storey window is seen
only as a nuisance, leading to the windows being nailed down with loss of
fresh air. It is difficult to face anxieties about suicide. Meanwhile, Ms
Poplar is overawed by the sociologist patient in the next bed who might
actually benefit more from a bit of help.

Ms Sycamore's cases (11)

Case no 3: woman with breast cancer and bony secondary
First reported 8th March, 1972. The problem of 'whether to tell' the patient
with cancer. And, if so, who should do it? What should Ms Sycamore do
when the patient says, 'I think the doctor believes I have cancer and doesn't
want to tell me'? There are bony secondaries and a pathological fracture
20 years after the original mastectomy for cancer.

Follow-up 8th June, 1972. The patient seems much more composed since
an orthopaedic surgeon, consulted in connection with the fracture, told her
that she had had cancer. Ms Sycamore remains impaled on the exact words
used by the surgeon and whatever precise nuance he was trying to convey.
The physiotherapist still cannot go an inch further than the way the doctor
has set it up − but she also cannot allow herself to clarify how he *has* set it
up.

Follow-up 22nd June, 1972. The patient is depressed again.

Case no 10: lady of 74: fractured neck of humerus and lower end of radius
Reported 28th March, 1972. The problem is that somehow the energy Ms
Sycamore is putting into the case seems out of all proportion. She suspects
that she is being cruel but also that, in some peculiar way, the patient likes
it. Anxieties about the pathos of old age have probably blocked more
appropriate professional curiosity about the case-history and how the
accident happened, which remains unknown. This is rather astonishing in
view of the unusual combination of fractures.

Case no 17: problems with a student
Reported 29th June, 1972. The student is troublesome and inept in her work. Staff prejudices, old-fashioned ideas and half-recognised impulses to keep juniors down all add to the difficulty in handling the problem. The temptation to 'sink people' may be very concrete and is not confined to examiners and teachers. There was an episode in which a student had placed a very small woman in the physiotherapy department pool with the water up over her nose.

Case no 19: man aged 74: above-knee amputation; chronic bronchitis and congestive heart failure ('Old Mr Carter')
First reported 6th July, 1972. There was an attempt (unsuccessful) at fitting an artificial limb. Ms Sycamore has to get him mobilised but the problem may really be to allow the poor fellow to die in peace. Some of the inappropriate struggling covers repressed hatred and contempt for a mutilated amputee.

Follow-up 13th July, 1972. The ward staff arrange his discharge without consulting Ms Sycamore and she feels slighted.

Follow-up 6th September, 1972. He is still there. When they finally get him standing up, he has a dripping anal sphincter. Defeat is now accepted but professional pride and optimism are wounded. (Compare Case 29 – 'Old Mr Hopkins'.)

Case no 22: a nurse: mobilisation after operation on knee
Reported 20th July, 1972. The knee was full of fibrous bands causing grindings and clickings. This is one of many discussions about quadriceps exercises. At first it is impossible to achieve anything and the muscles remain like blancmange, until, suddenly and mysteriously, they turn into a working unit. The patient's mother is a physiotherapist.

Case no 29: man aged 84: above-knee amputation; osteotomy at hip; colostomy; prostatectomy ('Old Mr Hopkins')
Reported 20th September, 1972. The amputation is for arterial disease and physiotherapy is to mobilise him and prepare him for use of an artificial limb. There are some similarities with another of her cases (Mr Carter) but this old man is much more engaging and arouses very different responses.

Case no 37: girl aged 19: physiotherapy student; meniscetomy
First reported 1st November, 1972. The present disability is now out of all proportion, her gait is bizarre. The principal of the physiotherapy school probably wants to get rid of her. Ms Sycamore is impeded by conflicting roles as therapist, teacher, and confidante. She has conflicting loyalties between the department and the patient and difficulties about confidentiality encourage evasion of any serious exploration of this girl's anxieties.

Follow-up 22nd November, 1972. Matters are getting worse. In spite of the gross and obvious disability and unsuitability of this girl as a physiotherapist, a cloak and dagger atmosphere is developing around the issue of confidentiality.

Follow-up 6th December, 1972. The Principal has dropped this girl from the school and Ms Sycamore is trying hard to get the girl to talk. The discussion exposes quite a lot about the expectations and attitudes of people entering the physiotherapy profession. It also exposes the ease with which it is possible to get oneself muddled up with one's patients. There are related problems as to recognition of physiotherapists' varying suitabilities for different aspects of the work and especially for this 'counselling' aspect of work with their students.

Case no 38: boy aged 18: a peculiar knee; ? compensation neurosis
First reported 8th November, 1972. A chaotic story of probable medical mismanagement for a couple of years and severe hysterical disability now. Manipulation under anaesthetic is followed by a 'maniac episode' lasting a couple of days.

Follow-up 22nd November, 1972. An interesting question as to why Ms Sycamore's students make much better progress with him than she does. A discussion of the dynamics and rival merits of their firm, tough techniques as contrasted with her gentle, seductive approaches whereby women may get men flat on their backs.

Case no 51: man aged 81: fractured shoulder, one year previously
First reported 17th January, 1973. He did very well then. Ms Sycamore is worried because she dislikes him heartily owing to an irritating pious complacency. This contrasts with the more usual dislike of patients who do badly. He has reappeared with what now appear to be psychological difficulties presenting as shoulder difficulties. There is not much indication for physiotherapy but Ms Sycamore is persisting as she senses that the treatment has a supportive function. The case involves discussion of some of the tactics that help therapists to stay with patients they dislike.

Follow-up 24th January, 1973. Ms Sycamore still dislikes the patient but feels less imprisoned following last week's discussion. As a result, she no longer has to keep popping out of the cubicle in her former compulsive way.

Follow-up 20th June, 1973. A telegraphic follow-up. The patient is being treated by somebody else now and Ms Sycamore is greeted, from a distance, as a long-lost friend. She is glad to leave it at that.

Case no 58: middle-aged woman: below-knee amputation
First reported 7th February, 1973. This was for severe recurrent cellulitis with septicaemia. The present problem is mobilisation and rehabilitation. The knee is impossible to straighten and Ms Sycamore is enraged at the critical attitude of the doctors to the physiotherapists' achievement or lack

of it. Manipulation under anaesthetic may help but the woman collapses each time for several days afterwards. Can anyone really forgive a surgeon who has amputated their leg?

Follow-up 4th April, 1973. More manipulations and moderate progress in the meantime. The surgeon has been to the USA and there is a frisson of excitement around his return and the impending discharge of the patient. The atmosphere seems full of unrealistic thinking about future plans and possibilities.

Follow-up 11th April, 1973. Ms Sycamore discovers ability to make better contact with the doctors instead of clinging to bad relations with them (like the patient's inability to give up the bad leg). The patient's difficulty in realistic adaptation to her future prosthesis is parallel, it is now revealed, to equal unreality in the physiotherapists (and doctors?). Thus, it seems almost tactless to ask what actually happened to the amputated leg and it emerges that several members of the group, including Ms Sycamore, have hardly ever seen an artificial one at close quarters.

Follow-up 9th May, 1973. The struggle towards establishing realistic aims continues. Patients and staff tend to find it equally difficult to accept the bony limitations to mobilisation of the knee. They also find it equally difficult to hear each other's messages.

Follow-up 20th June, 1973. There has been great progress with the final prosthesis but, unfortunately, new difficulties of a small sore which could get worse. Was the amputation high enough? More cold reality: nobody has thought of taking this woman on a bus although she is supposed to be resuming work as a schoolteacher in September. It seems that too much empathy may, in its way, be as blinding as too much professional detachment.

Follow-up 18th July, 1973. A retrospective view. Now the patient has been discharged. Ms Sycamore thinks this should have happened long ago and would have happened but for excessive preoccupation with the emotional problems which were reflected in dissension amongst the staff. Now there may be a psychiatric referral.

Case no 65: girl aged 14: removal of patella; hysteria
Reported 21st March, 1973. The background to the referral appears to be an incredible operation two years ago and surgical bungling ever since — but nobody can be very sure. There could be a self-respecting role for the physiotherapist, in treatment of hysterical disorders but they feel insulted and enraged unless (or even if?) the referral is dressed up and rationalised in physical terms.

Ms Teak's cases (11)

Case no 46: woman aged 42: backache; previous knee operations
Reported 13th December, 1972. Patient seems determined to have an operation *on her back* but the condition is not thought to have a physical cause. The doctors refer her for more physiotherapy *to the knees* and the physiotherapist bears the brunt of the resentment. The psychiatric consultant has already opted out of this case and the physiotherapist gets nowhere in her own attempt to discuss the patient's problems with her. The patient appears to be seeking some form of maltreatment so that soothing treatments, like ice-packs, may be particularly unsuitable. Should the physiotherapist seek one of her more unpleasant forms of treatment to satisfy this patient? The patient is a gym teacher. Is this too close to physiotherapy for comfort?

Cases nos 52 and 53: a pair of patients receiving pre-operative physiotherapy before very similar operations
Reported 17th January, 1973. She likes one of these patients and dislikes the other and expects to be lumbered with the one she dislikes for the next three months.

Follow-up 24th January, 1973. Following identical operations the man she disliked beforehand and thought would do badly has, in fact, done very well. On the other hand, the woman she liked is not doing very well and Ms Teak finds, to her surprise, that she has taken a sharp dislike to this woman and now feels quite pleasantly towards the man.

Case no 55: a young nurse: laminectomy and spinal fusion
First reported 24th January, 1973. A few days before the patient is due to be discharged home, Ms Teak discovers that this involves a five-hour rail journey. This leads on to learning about an illegitimate baby a few years ago, a nasty atmosphere at home and the present tangle of denial and secrecy. The patient has an unusual capacity to dissociate — to remain unaware of what she is doing and this fits all too well with the surgical ward where channels of communication are uncertain and a stiff upper lip is the favoured demeanour. Thus, the arrangements for convalence may get bungled. The patient is told how to take a bath but not whether she may make love or become pregnant. The physiotherapist, in whose mind this begins to dawn, does not know who to tell or what to say.

Follow-up 31st January, 1973. As if by magic, her troubles have disappeared and she is, once again, a cheerful resilient nurse while another girl, with a similar operation (Case 56) has become tearful and helpless instead. Reinstatement in the role of nurse seems to be more comfortable than suffering in the role of patient but there is a heavy price in loss of awareness and restriction of psychological experience.
   Something similar to this patient's psychopathology is possibly involved in a mental stance that enables hospital staff to switch their feelings and allegiances from patient to patient — and even, apparently, to enjoy the process, as they pass rapidly in and out of hospital. Is it also related to the

temperament of the patient who gets drunk at a party, wakes up pregnant, gives the baby into adoption — and appears to forget about it soon afterwards? How deep do all these appearances go?

Case no 56: girl of about 20: laminectomy, prolapsed inter-vertebral disc

First reported 24th January, 1973. The case is presented as a pair together with Case 55. She did not come into focus at this point and there appeared to be no particular trouble.

Follow-up 31st January, 1973. The next week roles have switched around and she is tearful and anxious whereas the other girl is ascendant. Belatedly, it is now recalled that, after a pre-operative enema, she went into a panic with over-breathing and tetany. This led to an extended discussion of how to manage disturbing procedures as well as the recognition that some procedures which may appear to be relatively 'neutral' may actually be experienced as dreadfully intimate assaults.

Case no 68: Ms Teak's discussion with the surgeon

Reported 4th April, 1973. This arose from her hunch that all cases of operation on the back are liable to be followed by depression. The discussion was about who should explain the nature of operations to patients beforehand and about how realistic warnings of pain should be? Behind this discussion of 'the management of pain' there appears to be some expectation that, as if by magic, pain ought to go away if only the correct frame of mind can be achieved. This may spring from the difficulty that hospital staff have in facing the reality of the pain their patients suffer. Much of the fear to prescribe analgesics is due to the insistent need to suppress awareness that people are suffering. Nevertheless there is a distinction between pain and distress and some discussion of what are the additional factors which turn pain into unbearable distress.

Case no 69: man: laminectomy and spinal fusion

Reported 9th May, 1973. The problem of a patient who keeps repeating the same questions about his treatment and prognosis. Hints of problems at home.

Case no 71: a sailor with an injured knee

Reported 16th May, 1973. The case is complicated and was originally treated abroad. Eventually he had an infected haematoma, a quadriceps transplant and a skin graft. Although nobody is to blame there is a lingering unease and some suspicion that the physiotherapist may have pulled the wound open. Beyond this we discover some tendency to feel responsible for everything that goes wrong. This may spring from some curious grandiosity; there may be secret triumph over the mistakes of colleagues and this is covered by self-accusation; there are problems of loyalties and idealisation of one's own group.

208

Case no 72: elderly woman: total replacement of hip joint
First reported 16th May, 1973. The prosthesis re-dislocated. The patient
should have been warned not to climb out of bed without a nurse. Why
does Ms Teak feel responsible?

Follow-up 23rd May, 1973. Are there other anxieties beyond questions of
relapse and litigation? Are family feelings involved? Probing can lead into
unexpected territory.

Follow-up 30th May, 1973. View of the case narrows down towards reassurance of a good prognosis as the only admissable issue.

Case no 77: man with a spinal fusion operation: he also has arthritic hips
Reported 30th May, 1973. The problem is that she describes him as 'batty'
and is afraid he will destroy the operation by bending his back before it is
safe to do so. Ms Teak had great difficulty in clarifying what she meant by
'batty' and her colleagues were doubtful about the reality of her fears about
the possible failure of the operation. There is some sense that 'batty' blind-
to-danger behaviour may spring from an effort to expel anxiety from oneself
into everybody else. Thus Ms Teak (for example) is full of anxiety about the
outcome of this case whilst the patient can carry on as if he is quite
unconcerned.

Ms Yew's cases (8)

Case no 40: boy aged 13: dying of polycystic disease
Reported 15th November, 1972. A few days before his death he said, 'I
can't stand much more of this'. The problem is not so much any question
of what staff can do for a distressed dying child who can hardly breathe.
The problem is more one of how to remain in close contact but not chatty,
not bustling about.

Case no 41: girl aged 14: cerebral palsy; tendon transplant
Reported 15th November, 1972. The problem is presented as an instance of
the over-protective mother. Her opposition to her daughter's necessary operation is suspected to spring from her own anxiety and hostility to the child.
After everybody else has failed, the surgeon surprises everybody by per-
suading her easily — whereupon, she talks of the impending admission to
hospital for the operation as a holiday for the girl.
  The physiotherapists seem to share something of the mother's wishful
fear that the surgeon be a frightening butcher and the mother's silly pretence
that the hospital is a holiday camp is not so very far from the chaotic
carnival atmosphere generated in many hospital departments by haphazard
organisation, rota systems that leave nobody in particular responsible and
so forth. Thus Ms Yew's own phraseology as she remarks, in passing, that
she would 'be quite happy to trot along to the surgeon' if necessary.

Case no 49: girl aged 3: astrocytoma

Reported 20th December, 1972. The condition was not operable but she is doing reasonably well after radiotherapy. There is good progress but curious problems of shouting during her treatment and sudden collapses into 'feeling poorly'. Ms Yew is familiar with hypochondria and anxiety in little children but the others, inexperienced in this work, find it harder to imagine and try to see more of the anxiety as being 'really' in the parents.

Then the appalling history comes out. These parents have already lost two other children, one from gastroenteritis and another from spina bifida. Thus, the unacknowledged hospital maxim is reinforced — beware of going into things! It is always best not to ask and not to know. No one is surprised that Ms Yew has remained carefully vague about the actual prognosis for the case.

Case no 54: girl aged 2: neo-natal meningitis; amentia; quadriplegia

Reported 17th January, 1973. The child is a complete vegetable in residential institutional care and the mother is afraid she would murder her if she has her home. She is a simple Welsh woman with an absentee Jamaican father to her baby. Ms Yew was urged by her colleagues to present the case to the seminar.

This is not a case for physiotherapy and neither is it a case in which the woman should be 'helped' to take the child home. On the contrary, she requires help to detach herself from what is virtually a stillbirth and she should not be pushed into sharing an inappropriate medical ethic about struggling on with treatment until death. The physiotherapists may best help this woman by learning to say, 'No' to the doctors referring the case.

An important issue here is the recognition of what type of referrals you are getting: when they are referred because you are idealised and, conversely, (or indeed simultaneously) when the aim is to crush you under the impossible. Idealisation often veils hostility.

Case no 74: a small child with pathological fracture

Reported 16th May, 1973. She was following instructions to continue a routine of exercises for somebody else's patient. Owing to the presence of a rare bone disease it seems that she broke the leg although neither she nor the child were aware, at the time, that anything unusual had happened. It was noticed some hours later. It was obviously not her fault but unpleasant feelings are generated.

Case no 75: a boy: congenital malformation

Reported 23rd May, 1973. He is moderately disabled. Malformation was caused by maternal rubella during pregnancy. The boy complains that it is 'not my fault' but evidently feels that it is somebody's fault.

Case no 76: a boy: disability after road accident

Reported 23rd May, 1973. There appears to be no physical injury but he has considerable residual disability of psychogenic nature. He has a peculiar gait and walks with floppy feet in the hospital. At home he is severely

210

disabled, refusing to walk. Father is known to be an alcoholic and there is serious family disruption. The referral to the physiotherapy department seems to be a supportive measure in which nobody believes.

Case no 78: baby boy aged two: arthrogryphosis – litigation
Reported 13th June, 1973. A rare, crippling congenital disorder requiring various operations and physiotherapy. Parents are sueing another hospital where mother had appendicectomy during pregnancy. The problem is Ms Yew's feeling that she 'ducked out of it' in referring the mother to discuss her anxieties with the surgeon whereas it should have been possible to do better than that.